# BALANCE YOUR
# BLOOD SUGAR

## An Insulin Resistance Diet Plan And Cookbook For Health And Happiness

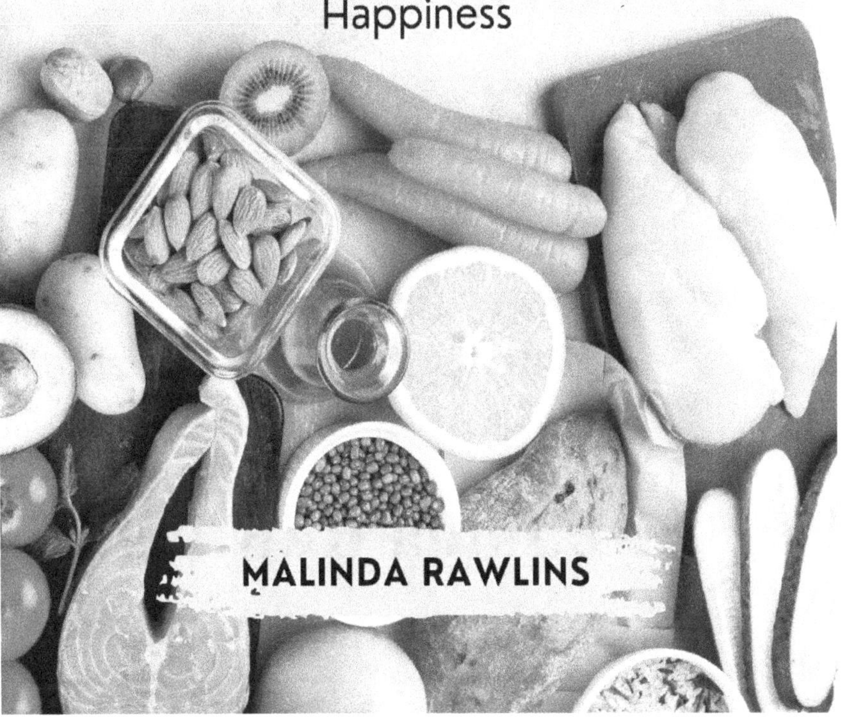

# Balance Your Blood Sugar

An Insulin resistance Diet Plan and Cookbook for Health and Happiness

BY

## Malinda Rawlins

# Disclaimer

This book is not intended to diagnose, treat, or cure any medical condition. It is intended for informational and educational purposes only. The information contained in this book should not be used to replace the advice of a qualified healthcare professional. Please consult with your healthcare provider before making any changes to your exercise routine or diet plan. The authors and publisher of this book are not responsible for any adverse effects or consequences resulting from the use of the information contained in this book. The recipes included in this book may not be suitable for everyone, and it is the responsibility of the reader to determine their suitability for their individual needs. The authors and publisher of this book do not assume any liability for the use or misuse of the information contained in this book.

You are responsible for your actions by acting on the thought and views shared in this book.

You are encouraged to print this book for easy reading.

# Table of Contents

# Why This Book?

Are you tired of feeling sluggish, irritable, and unable to focus because of blood sugar imbalances? Are you struggling to manage your insulin resistance or diabetes? If so, "Balance Your Blood Sugar: An Insulin resistance Diet Plan and Cookbook for Health and Happiness" is the right book for you.

This book is designed to help you take control of your health and improve your quality of life through diet and lifestyle changes. It provides practical, science-based strategies for managing insulin resistance and optimizing blood sugar levels, as well as delicious, low-glycemic recipes that will help you feel satisfied and nourished.

But this book is about more than just managing a medical condition. It's about finding balance and feeling your best every day. It's about taking charge of your health and finding joy in nourishing your body with wholesome, delicious food.

With "Balance Your Blood Sugar," you'll learn:

- The science behind insulin resistance and blood sugar imbalances
- Simple, practical strategies for managing insulin resistance and optimizing blood sugar levels
- Delicious, low-glycemic recipes that will help you feel satisfied and nourished
- Valuable tips for incorporating healthy habits into your daily routine
- And much more!

Whether you're looking to manage your insulin resistance or diabetes or simply want to feel your best and improve your overall health, "Balance Your Blood Sugar" has something for you.

So don't wait — take charge of your health and start feeling your best today with this comprehensive guide to managing insulin resistance and optimizing blood sugar levels.

# Chapter 1

## The ABCs of Insulin resistance

nsulin resistance is a complex issue that can have significant impacts on the body and overall health. Understanding the ABCs of insulin resistance can help you better manage this condition and reduce the risk of associated complications.

A is for "abnormal blood sugar levels." Insulin resistance is characterized by high blood sugar levels, which can cause a range of symptoms such as fatigue, irritability, and difficulty concentrating. High blood sugar levels can result in serious, long-term issues, including damage to the nerves, kidneys, and eyes.

B is for "body weight." Insulin resistance can contribute to weight gain and obesity, as the body's cells are not able to effectively use glucose (sugar) for energy. Instead, the body stores excess glucose as fat, leading to weight gain. Maintaining a healthy body weight through weight loss can improve insulin sensitivity and decrease the possibility of insulin resistance.

C is for "complications." Insulin resistance can lead to a higher likelihood of experiencing other health problems, such as heart disease, stroke, and high blood pressure. It can also lead to the development of type 2 diabetes, a disorder characterized by the body's inability to maintain normal blood sugar levels. Managing insulin resistance through diet and lifestyle changes can help reduce the risk of these complications.

Understanding the ABCs of insulin resistance is an essential step in managing this condition and improving your overall health. By making diet and lifestyle changes, working with a healthcare provider, and monitoring blood sugar levels, you can effectively manage insulin resistance and reduce the risk of associated complications.

# What is insulin resistance?

Insulin resistance is a state in which the cells of the body do not respond appropriately to insulin, a hormone produced by the pancreas that helps to control blood sugar levels. As a result, the body needs to produce more insulin to keep blood sugar levels in check, which can eventually lead to high insulin levels and the development of insulin resistance.

Insulin resistance is often associated with conditions such as type 2 diabetes, prediabetes, and metabolic syndrome. An increased risk of other health issues, including heart disease, stroke, and high blood pressure, are also linked to it.

Insulin resistance can be caused by being overweight or obese, having a family history of insulin resistance or type 2 diabetes, leading a sedentary lifestyle, having high blood pressure, having high levels of triglycerides in the blood, and having low levels of HDL cholesterol in the blood.

Certain groups of people, such as women with polycystic ovary syndrome (PCOS), people of certain ethnicities, and older adults, may also be at increased risk of developing insulin resistance. Managing insulin resistance through diet and lifestyle changes can also assist in the prevention of insulin resistance and its associated complications.

It is also essential to work with a healthcare provider to monitor blood sugar levels and make any necessary changes to diet and medication.

## How does it affect the body?

Insulin resistance can affect the body in a number of ways. First and foremost, it can lead to high blood sugar levels, which can cause a range of symptoms such as fatigue, irritability, and difficulty concentrating. High blood sugar levels can also lead to long-term complications such as nerve damage and kidney damage, and eye damage.

Insulin resistance can also contribute to weight gain and obesity, as the body's cells are not able to effectively use glucose (sugar) for energy. Instead, the body stores excess glucose as fat, leading to weight gain. This can be a vicious cycle, as excess weight can further exacerbate insulin resistance and make it even more challenging to manage.

In addition, insulin resistance is associated with an increased risk of developing other health complications, which include heart disease, stroke, and high blood pressure. Insulin resistance can also lead to the development of type 2 diabetes, a condition that causes the body to be unable to properly regulate blood sugar levels.

Managing insulin resistance through diet and making alterations to one's lifestyle, such as consuming a nutritious diet and participating in regular physical activity, and maintaining a healthy weight, can help reduce the risk of developing these complications. It is also essential to work with a healthcare provider to monitor blood sugar levels and make any necessary changes to diet and medication. By taking steps to manage insulin resistance, you can improve your overall health and reduce the risk of long-term complications.

# Risk factors and complications

There are various risk factors that can increase the likelihood of developing insulin resistance, including:

- Being overweight or obese: Excess weight, particularly abdominal fat, can increase the risk of insulin resistance. Losing weight and maintaining a healthy body weight can help improve insulin sensitivity and decrease the risk of insulin resistance.

- Having a family history of insulin resistance or type 2 diabetes: If you have a family history of these conditions, you may be at increased risk of developing insulin resistance yourself.

- Leading a sedentary lifestyle: Regular physical activity can help improve insulin sensitivity and reduce the risk of insulin resistance.

- Having high blood pressure: High blood pressure is a risk factor for insulin resistance and can also be a complication of insulin resistance.

- Having high levels of triglycerides in the blood: Triglycerides are a type of fat that can contribute to insulin resistance.

- Having low levels of HDL cholesterol in the blood: HDL cholesterol, also known as the "good" cholesterol, helps remove excess cholesterol from the body. Low levels of HDL cholesterol can increase the risk of insulin resistance.

In addition to the risk factors listed above, certain groups of people may be more likely to develop insulin resistance, including:

- Women with polycystic ovary syndrome (PCOS): PCOS is a condition that affects hormones and can increase the risk of insulin resistance.

- People of certain ethnicities: African Americans, Hispanic Americans, and Native Americans, are at increased risk of insulin resistance and type 2 diabetes.

- Older adults: As we age, our bodies become less sensitive to insulin, which can increase the risk of insulin resistance.

The complications of insulin resistance can be severe and include an increased risk of developing type 2 diabetes, heart disease, stroke, and high blood pressure. It is essential to take steps to manage insulin resistance and reduce the risk of these complications.

Managing insulin resistance through diet and lifestyle changes, such as eating a healthy diet, getting regular physical activity, and maintaining a healthy weight, can help reduce the risk of developing insulin resistance and its associated complications. It is also essential to work with a healthcare provider to monitor blood sugar levels and make any necessary changes to diet and medication. By taking an active role in managing your health, you can reduce the risk of insulin resistance and its associated complications and improve your overall quality of life.

# Chapter 2

## A Low-Glycemic Diet to the Rescue

nsulin resistance can be effectively managed through diet and lifestyle changes, such as following a low-glycemic diet. A low-glycemic diet is a type of eating plan that emphasizes foods that are low on the glycemic index (GI), which is a ranking system that assesses the effect of various kinds of carbohydrates on blood sugar levels. Foods with a low GI value are absorbed more slowly by the body, which helps to keep blood

sugar levels stable and reduces the risk of insulin resistance.

# What is a low-glycemic diet?

A low-glycemic diet is based on the concept of the glycemic index (GI), which ranks carbohydrates based on their impact on blood sugar levels. Foods that have a high glycemic index (GI) are rapidly absorbed by the body and may cause a sudden increase in blood sugar levels. Conversely, foods with a low GI are absorbed more slowly, resulting in a slower and more gradual impact on blood sugar levels.

Low-glycemic foods are typically high in fiber and other nutrients, and they are absorbed more slowly by the body, which helps to keep blood sugar levels stable. This can be particularly beneficial for people with insulin resistance, as it helps to reduce the risk of high blood sugar levels and the associated complications.

Low-glycemic foods include:

- Fruits and vegetables: Most fruits and vegetables are low on the glycemic index, with the exception of some starchy vegetables such as potatoes and corn.

- Whole grains: Whole grains, such as oats, quinoa, and brown rice, are high in fiber and have a low GI value.

- Legumes: Legumes, such as beans, lentils, and chickpeas, are low on the glycemic index and are a good source of protein and fiber.

- Nuts and seeds: Nuts and seeds, such as almonds, walnuts, and chia seeds, are low on the glycemic index and are a good source of healthy fats and fiber.

- Lean protein sources: Lean protein sources, such as chicken, fish, and tofu, are low on the glycemic index and can help keep blood sugar levels stable.

In addition to the foods listed above, it is crucial to limit or avoid foods that are high on the glycemic index, such as white bread, pasta, and sugary snacks. These foods are absorbed quickly by the body and can cause a rapid increase in blood sugar levels, which can contribute to insulin resistance.

Following a low-glycemic diet can be an effective way to manage insulin resistance and improve blood sugar control. It is essential to work with a healthcare provider and a registered dietitian to develop an eating plan that is right for you and meets your individual needs and goals. With the right plan in place, you can take control of your health and manage insulin resistance effectively.

# The benefits of a low-glycemic diet

A low-glycemic diet is an eating plan that emphasizes foods that are low on the glycemic index (GI), a ranking system that assesses the effect of various kinds of carbohydrates on blood sugar levels. Foods with a low GI value are absorbed more slowly by the body, which helps to keep blood sugar levels stable and reduces the risk of insulin resistance. There are numerous benefits to following a low-glycemic diet, including:

- Improved blood sugar control: One of the primary benefits of a low-glycemic diet is improved blood sugar control. By choosing foods that are absorbed slowly by the body, you can help keep blood sugar levels stable, which can be especially beneficial for people with insulin resistance or other conditions that affect blood sugar control.

- Weight loss: A low-glycemic diet can also be helpful for weight loss. Because low-glycemic foods are absorbed more slowly by the body, they can help keep you feeling full and satisfied, which can help you eat less and lose weight. In addition, low-glycemic foods are often lower in calories and higher in fiber, which can also contribute to weight loss.

- Reduced risk of type 2 diabetes: Following a low-glycemic diet has been shown to be beneficial for people with prediabetes or at risk of developing type 2 diabetes. By keeping blood sugar levels stable, a low-glycemic diet can help reduce the risk of developing type 2 diabetes.

- Improved heart health: There is some evidence to suggest that following a low-glycemic diet can help improve heart health. A low-glycemic diet can help lower blood pressure, reduce cholesterol levels, and reduce the risk of heart disease.

- Increased energy levels: By keeping blood sugar levels stable, a low-glycemic diet can help improve energy levels and reduce feelings of fatigue.

- Improved mood: Some studies have found that following a low-glycemic diet can improve mood and reduce feelings of anxiety and depression.

In addition to the benefits listed above, following a low-glycemic diet can also help reduce the risk of other health problems, such as kidney disease, nerve damage, and eye damage.

It is important to note that a low-glycemic diet is not a one-size-fits-all solution, and it is essential to work with a healthcare provider and a registered dietitian to develop an eating plan that is right for you and meets your individual needs and goals. In general, a low-glycemic diet should include a variety of foods, including fruits and vegetables, whole grains, legumes, nuts and seeds, and lean protein sources. It is also important to limit or avoid foods that are high on the glycemic index, such as white bread, pasta, and sugary snacks.

In addition to following a low-glycemic diet, other lifestyle changes, such as getting regular physical activity and maintaining a healthy weight, can help improve insulin sensitivity and reduce the risk of insulin resistance. By taking a holistic approach to your health and making the necessary changes to your diet and lifestyle, you can effectively manage insulin resistance and improve your overall quality of life.

# How to incorporate low-glycemic foods into your meals

Incorporating low-glycemic foods into your meals is an effective way to manage insulin resistance and improve blood sugar control. Here are some tips for adding more low-glycemic foods to your diet:

- Choose whole grains: Instead of white bread, pasta, and rice, opt for whole grains such as oats, quinoa, and brown rice. These are lower on the glycemic index and are a good source of fiber, which can help keep you feeling full and satisfied.

- Eat more fruits and vegetables: Fruits and vegetables are generally low on the glycemic index and are a good source of fiber, vitamins, and minerals. Aim at filling a portion of your plate with vegetables and fruits at every meal.

- Include legumes in your meals: Legumes, such as beans, lentils, and chickpeas, are low on the glycemic index and are a good source of protein and fiber. Add them to soups, stews, and salads, or use them as a replacement for meat in dishes like tacos and chili.

- Snack on nuts and seeds: Nuts and seeds, such as almonds, walnuts, and chia seeds, are low on the glycemic index and are a good source of healthy fats and fiber. Keep a bag of nuts or seeds on hand for a quick and healthy snack.

- Choose lean protein sources: Lean protein sources, such as chicken, fish, and tofu, are low on the glycemic index and can help keep blood sugar levels stable. Include a serving of protein in every meal and snack.

Incorporating low-glycemic foods into your meals is just one aspect of managing insulin resistance. It is also essential to work with a healthcare provider and a registered dietitian to develop an eating plan that is right for you and meets your individual needs and goals. In addition, getting regular physical activity, maintaining a healthy weight, and managing stress can all help improve insulin sensitivity and reduce the risk of insulin resistance.

Here are some additional tips for incorporating low-glycemic foods into your meals:

- Plan ahead: Planning your meals and snacks in advance can help ensure that you have a variety of low-glycemic foods on hand. Make a grocery list of low-glycemic foods and stick to it when shopping.

- Keep it simple: You don't have to make complicated or time-consuming meals to incorporate low-glycemic foods into your diet. Simply choosing whole grains instead of refined grains, adding more vegetables to your meals, and snacking on nuts and seeds can make a big difference.

- Be mindful of portion sizes: Even low-glycemic foods can cause blood sugar levels to rise if eaten in large quantities. Be mindful of portion sizes and aim to consume reasonable amounts of all types of foods.

- Get creative: There are plenty of delicious and creative ways to incorporate low-glycemic foods into your meals. Try adding nuts and seeds to salads, making a stir-fry with a variety of vegetables and lean protein, or using beans as a base for a hearty soup.

By following these tips and working with a healthcare provider and a registered dietitian, you can effectively incorporate low-glycemic foods into your meals and improve your overall health. By making changes to your diet and lifestyle, you can take control of your health and manage insulin resistance effectively.

# Chapter 3

## Simple Strategies for Optimal Blood Sugar Control

Maintaining optimal blood sugar control is an important part of managing insulin resistance and reducing the risk of related conditions such as type 2 diabetes and metabolic syndrome. There are several simple strategies that individuals with insulin resistance can use to help improve blood sugar control and improve their overall health.

One key strategy for optimal blood sugar control is to focus on eating a healthy diet that is rich in fiber, protein, and healthy fats and that limits the intake of refined carbohydrates and added sugars. This can help improve insulin sensitivity and better regulate blood sugar levels. It is also important to pay attention to portion sizes, as eating too much of any type of food can contribute to weight gain and difficulty managing blood sugar levels.

Increasing physical activity is another important strategy for optimal blood sugar control. Regular physical activity can help improve insulin sensitivity, burn excess calories, and reduce the risk of developing chronic conditions such as heart disease and type 2 diabetes. Aim for at least 150 minutes of moderate-intensity physical activity per week or 75 minutes of vigorous-intensity activity.

In addition to diet and exercise, there are several other simple strategies that individuals with insulin resistance can use to help improve blood sugar control. These include:

- Monitoring blood sugar levels: Regularly monitoring blood sugar levels can help individuals with insulin resistance identify patterns and trends and make necessary adjustments to their diet and lifestyle in order to better manage blood sugar levels.

- Staying hydrated: Drinking plenty of water and staying hydrated can help regulate blood sugar levels and improve insulin sensitivity. Aim for at least 8-8 ounces of water per day, and limit intake of sugary drinks and alcohol.

- Getting enough sleep: Adequate sleep is important for overall health, and it can also help improve insulin sensitivity and blood sugar control. Aim for 7-9 hours of sleep per night.

- Managing stress: Chronic stress can interfere with blood sugar control and increase the risk of insulin resistance. Managing stress through activities such as meditation, yoga, and exercise can help improve insulin sensitivity and better regulate blood sugar levels.

- Limiting alcohol intake: While moderate alcohol intake may have some health benefits, excessive alcohol consumption can contribute to weight gain and increase the risk of insulin resistance. It is important to limit alcohol intake to no more than one drink per day for women and two drinks per day for men.

- Seeking support: It can be helpful to seek support from a healthcare team, a registered dietitian, or a support group as you make changes to your diet and lifestyle to manage insulin resistance and improve blood sugar control.

Overall, there are several simple strategies that individuals with insulin resistance can use to help improve blood sugar control and improve their overall health. By following a healthy diet, increasing physical activity, monitoring blood sugar levels, staying hydrated, getting enough sleep, managing stress, and seeking support, individuals with insulin resistance can take control of their health and reduce their risk of developing related conditions such as type 2 diabetes and metabolic syndrome.

# Tips for managing insulin resistance through diet and lifestyle changes

Managing insulin resistance through diet and lifestyle changes is an important step in improving your overall health and reducing the risk of associated complications. Here are some tips for managing insulin resistance through diet and lifestyle changes:

- Eat a healthy diet: A healthy diet is an important aspect of managing insulin resistance. Choose foods that are low on the glycemic index, such as fruits and vegetables, whole grains, legumes, nuts and seeds, and lean protein sources. Limit or avoid foods that are high on the glycemic index, such as white bread, pasta, and sugary snacks.

- Get regular physical activity: Regular physical activity can help improve insulin sensitivity and reduce the risk of insulin resistance. The goal should be to engage in at least 150 minutes of moderate-intensity physical activity or 75 minutes of vigorous-intensity exercise on a weekly basis.

- Maintain a healthy weight: Excess weight, particularly abdominal fat, can increase the risk of insulin resistance. Losing weight and maintaining a healthy body weight can help improve insulin sensitivity and reduce the risk of insulin resistance.

- Monitor blood sugar levels: Working with a healthcare provider to monitor blood sugar levels is an important aspect of managing insulin resistance. By keeping track of your blood sugar levels, you can identify any patterns or problems and make any necessary changes to your diet or medication.

- Manage stress: Stress can increase the risk of insulin resistance. Finding ways to manage stress, such as relaxation techniques, exercise, or therapy, can help improve insulin sensitivity and reduce the risk of insulin resistance.

- Get enough sleep: Getting enough sleep is important for overall health, including insulin sensitivity. Aim for 7-9 hours of sleep per night to help improve insulin sensitivity and reduce the risk of insulin resistance.

- Don't smoke: Smoking can increase the risk of insulin resistance. If you smoke, consider quitting to improve insulin sensitivity and reduce the risk of insulin resistance.

By following these tips and working with a healthcare provider, you can effectively manage insulin resistance through diet and lifestyle changes and improve your overall health. By taking an active role in managing your health, you can reduce the risk of insulin resistance and its associated complications and improve your overall quality of life.

# The importance of regular physical activity

Regular physical activity is an important aspect of managing insulin resistance and improving overall health. Physical activity helps improve insulin sensitivity and reduce the risk of insulin resistance, as well as a number of other health benefits.

One of the primary benefits of regular physical activity is its ability to improve insulin sensitivity. Insulin sensitivity refers to the body's ability to use insulin effectively to regulate blood sugar levels. When the body is insulin sensitive, it can use glucose (sugar) for energy more efficiently, which helps to keep blood sugar levels stable and reduces the risk of insulin resistance. Regular physical activity can help improve insulin sensitivity, which can be especially beneficial for people with insulin resistance or other conditions that affect blood sugar control.

In addition to its effects on insulin sensitivity, regular physical activity has a number of other health benefits. It can help improve cardiovascular health, reduce the risk of heart disease, lower blood pressure, and improve cholesterol levels. Physical activity can also help with weight loss and maintenance, as it helps to burn calories and increase muscle mass.

Regular physical activity can also have mental health benefits, such as reducing stress, improving mood, and increasing energy levels. It can also help to improve sleep quality, which is important for overall health.

Incorporating regular physical activity into your routine can be challenging, but it is worth the effort. Aim for at least 30 minutes of moderate-intensity physical activity most days of the week or at least 150 minutes per week. Moderate-intensity activity includes activities such as brisk walking, swimming, and cycling. If you are new to physical activity or have medical conditions, it is important to talk to your healthcare provider before starting a new exercise routine.

There are many different ways to get regular physical activity, and the key is to find activities that you enjoy and that fit into your lifestyle. Some options might include walking or biking for transportation, joining a sports team or club, or taking up a new hobby such as dancing or yoga.

In conclusion, regular physical activity is an important aspect of managing insulin resistance and improving overall health. By incorporating physical activity into your routine, you can take control of your health and improve your insulin sensitivity, as well as enjoy a number of other health benefits.

# Strategies for reducing stress and improving sleep

Stress and sleep are important factors that can impact insulin resistance and overall health. Reducing stress and improving sleep can help improve insulin sensitivity and reduce the risk of insulin resistance. Here are some strategies for reducing stress and improving sleep:

- Practice relaxation techniques: Relaxation techniques, such as deep breathing, progressive muscle relaxation, and meditation, can help reduce stress and improve sleep. Set aside time each day to practice relaxation techniques to help manage stress and improve sleep.

- Exercise regularly: Exercise is a great way to reduce stress and improve sleep. Try to incorporate at least 30 minutes of moderate-intensity physical activity, like brisk walking or cycling, into your routine on most days of the week.

- Get enough sleep: Getting enough sleep is important for both physical and mental health. Try to get between 7 and

9 hours of sleep each night, and establish a regular sleep routine in order to enhance the quality of your sleep.

- Practice good sleep hygiene: Good sleep hygiene involves making changes to your sleep environment and habits to improve sleep. Some tips for good sleep hygiene include keeping a regular sleep schedule, avoiding caffeine and alcohol close to bedtime, and creating a comfortable sleep environment.

- Seek professional help: If you are struggling with stress or sleep problems, seeking help from a healthcare provider or mental health professional can be beneficial. They can provide support and guidance to help you manage stress and improve sleep.

By implementing these strategies, you can take steps to reduce stress and improve sleep, which can help improve insulin sensitivity and reduce the risk of insulin resistance. Remember that managing stress and sleep are ongoing processes, and it is important to be consistent and make these changes a part of your

daily routine to see lasting results.

# Chapter 4

## Meal Planning Made Easy

n this chapter, we will discuss the importance of meal planning for managing insulin resistance and improving overall health. We will cover the basics of meal planning, including understanding the role of carbohydrates, considering portion sizes, and planning for both meals and snacks. We will also provide tips for making meal planning easy, such as starting with a list of your favorite low-glycemic foods, using a meal planning template or app, and keeping it simple. By following the tips in this chapter, you can effectively manage insulin resistance and improve your overall health through meal planning.

# The basics of meal planning for insulin resistance

Meal planning can be an effective tool for managing insulin resistance and improving overall health. By planning your meals in advance, you can ensure that you are eating a balanced diet that includes a variety of low-glycemic foods, which can help keep blood sugar levels stable and reduce the risk of insulin resistance. Here are the basics of meal planning for insulin resistance:

- Know your goals: Before you start meal planning, it is important to know your goals. Do you want to lose weight, improve blood sugar control, or reduce the risk of insulin resistance? Knowing your goals will help you plan meals that meet your specific needs and goals.

- Understand the role of carbohydrates: Carbohydrates are a key component of a healthy diet, but they can also impact blood sugar levels. It is important to choose carbohydrates that are low on the glycemic index, as these are absorbed more slowly by the body and can help keep blood sugar levels stable. Low-glycemic foods include fruits and vegetables, whole grains, legumes, nuts and seeds, and lean protein sources.

- Consider portion sizes: Portion sizes are important when it comes to managing insulin resistance. Aim for reasonable portion sizes of all types of foods, including carbohydrates.

- Plan for meals and snacks: It is important to plan for both meals and snacks when meal planning for insulin resistance. This will help ensure that you are eating consistently throughout the day and keeping blood sugar levels stable.

- Be flexible: Meal planning does not have to be rigid. It is okay to make changes to your plan as needed, such as if you have a change in schedule or if you are craving a specific food. Just be sure to make healthy choices and stay within your goals.

- Keep it simple: You don't have to make complicated or time-consuming meals to plan your meals effectively. Simply choosing whole grains instead of refined grains, adding more vegetables to your meals, and snacking on nuts and seeds can make a big difference.

- Work with a healthcare provider and registered dietitian: It is important to work with a healthcare provider and a registered dietitian to develop an eating plan that is right for you and meets your individual needs and goals. They can provide guidance and support to help you manage insulin resistance effectively.

By following these tips and being consistent with your meal planning, you can effectively manage insulin resistance and improve your overall health. Remember to also consider other lifestyle factors, such as getting regular physical activity and reducing stress, which can also help improve insulin sensitivity and reduce the risk of insulin resistance.

## Grocery shopping tips and pantry staples

Grocery shopping and maintaining a well-stocked pantry are important aspects of managing insulin resistance and improving overall health. By making smart food choices at the grocery store and having a variety of healthy pantry staples on hand, you can effectively manage your diet and make it easier to stick to your meal plan. Here are some tips for grocery shopping and pantry staples for insulin resistance:

- Make a grocery list: Before you head to the grocery store, make a list of the low-glycemic foods you need for the week. This can help you stay organized and avoid impulse purchases.

- Shop the perimeter of the store: The perimeter of the grocery store is usually where the fresh produce, meats, and dairy products are located. These are generally lower on the glycemic index and are a good choice for insulin resistance.

- Don't shop when you're hungry: It is easier to make healthy food choices when you are not hungry. Try to shop when you are well-fed and have a clear mind.

- Read labels: Reading food labels can help you make informed decisions about what to buy. Look for foods that are low in added sugars and have a low glycemic index.

- Keep your pantry stocked with healthy staples: Having a variety of healthy pantry staples on hand can make it easier to stick to your meal plan. Some healthy pantry staples for insulin resistance include whole grains, such as oats and quinoa, legumes, such as beans and lentils, and nuts and seeds.

- Stock up on low-glycemic fruits and vegetables: Fresh fruits and vegetables are generally low on the glycemic index and are a good choice for insulin resistance. Keep your pantry stocked with a variety of frozen or canned low-glycemic fruits and vegetables, as well as fresh produce.

- Choose lean protein sources: Lean protein sources, such as chicken, fish, and tofu, are low on the glycemic index and can help keep blood sugar levels stable. Keep your pantry stocked with a variety of lean protein sources.

- Keep healthy snacks on hand: Having healthy snacks on hand can help prevent you from reaching for less healthy options when hunger strikes. Some healthy snack ideas for insulin resistance include nuts and seeds, fruit, and low-fat cheese.

By following these tips and being consistent with your grocery shopping and pantry staples, you can effectively manage insulin resistance and improve your overall health. Remember to work with a healthcare provider and a registered dietitian to develop an eating plan that is right for you and meets your individual needs and goals.

# Delicious, low-glycemic recipes for breakfast, lunch, dinner, and snacks

Eating a diet that is low in glycemic index (GI) is an effective way to manage insulin resistance and improve blood sugar control. Here are some delicious, low-glycemic recipes for breakfast, lunch, dinner, and snacks:

**Breakfast:**

- Overnight oats: Mix together rolled oats, milk or yogurt, fruit, and a dash of cinnamon. Let it sit in the refrigerator overnight, and enjoy it in the morning.

- Avocado toast: Spread mashed avocado on top of whole grain toast and top with a sprinkle of salt and pepper. Add a fried egg for extra protein.

- Banana smoothie: Blend together a banana, milk, or yogurt, a handful of spinach, and a scoop of protein powder for a quick and easy breakfast smoothie.

**Lunch:**

- Quinoa and black bean salad: Mix together cooked quinoa, black beans, diced tomatoes, corn, diced bell pepper, and chopped cilantro. Serve with a squeeze of lime juice and a sprinkle of chili flakes.

- Turkey and avocado wrap: Spread mashed avocado on a whole-grain wrap and top with sliced turkey, lettuce, and tomato. Roll it up and enjoy.

- Lentil soup: Sauté onions and carrots in a pot, then add in lentils, broth, and spices. Bring to a boil and let simmer until the lentils are cooked. Serve with a side of whole-grain bread.

**Dinner:**

- Grilled chicken and vegetable skewers: Thread chicken breasts and a variety of vegetables onto skewers and grill until the chicken is cooked through. Serve with a side of quinoa or brown rice.

- Chili: Sauté onions, peppers, and ground turkey in a pot. Add in canned tomatoes, kidney beans, and spices. Let simmer for 20-30 minutes and serve with a side of cornbread.

- Grilled salmon and roasted vegetables: Grill salmon fillets and roast a variety of vegetables in the oven. Serve with a side of quinoa or brown rice.

**Snacks:**

- Apple slices with almond butter: Slice an apple and spread with a spoonful of almond butter.

- Hummus and veggies: Dip sliced vegetables, such as bell peppers, carrots, and cucumbers, into a container of hummus.

- Greek yogurt with berries: Top a cup of Greek yogurt with a handful of fresh berries for a protein-packed snack.

By incorporating these low-glycemic recipes into your diet, you can effectively manage insulin resistance and improve your overall health. Remember to work with a healthcare provider and a registered dietitian to develop an eating plan that is right for you and meets your individual needs and goals. In addition to following a low-glycemic diet, other lifestyle changes, such as getting regular physical activity and maintaining a healthy weight, can also help improve insulin sensitivity and reduce the risk of insulin resistance.

Here are a few additional low-glycemic recipes to try:

- Baked sweet potato and black bean burritos: Stuff a whole grain tortilla with baked sweet potato, black beans, diced tomatoes, and cheese. Roll it up and bake in the oven until the cheese is melted.

- Veggie stir-fry: Sauté a variety of vegetables, such as bell peppers, onions, and carrots, in a pan with a little oil. Add tofu or lean protein of your choice and serve over quinoa or brown rice.

- Grilled eggplant and zucchini pasta: Slice eggplant and zucchini into thin rounds and grill until tender. Toss with cooked pasta, a jar of marinara sauce, and a sprinkle of Parmesan cheese.

By incorporating these low-glycemic recipes into your diet, you can effectively manage insulin resistance and improve your overall health. Remember to work with a healthcare provider and a registered dietitian to develop an eating plan that is right for you and meets your individual needs and goals. In addition to following a low-glycemic diet, other lifestyle changes, such as getting regular physical activity and maintaining a healthy weight, can also help improve insulin sensitivity and reduce the risk of insulin resistance.

# Chapter 5

## Staying on Track

n this chapter, we will explore strategies for sticking to your insulin resistance diet plan and maintaining progress over the long term. Adopting a new way of eating can be challenging, but with the right mindset and tools, you can successfully manage insulin resistance and improve your overall health. In this chapter, we will discuss strategies for overcoming common challenges, such as cravings and setbacks, and ways to stay motivated and on track. We will also discuss the importance of self-care and how it can help you. By the end of this chapter, you will have the knowledge and tools you need to stay on track and succeed on your insulin resistance diet plan.

## Strategies for maintaining progress and preventing relapse

Maintaining progress and preventing relapse are important considerations when following an insulin resistance diet plan. Here are some strategies for maintaining progress and preventing relapse:

- Set specific, achievable goals: Setting specific, achievable goals can help you stay focused and motivated. Consider setting short-term and long-term goals, and track your progress regularly.

- Create a supportive environment: Surrounding yourself with supportive people, such as friends and family, can help you stay committed to your health goals. Consider enlisting the support of a friend or family member to help you stay on track.

- Seek professional help: If you are struggling to maintain progress or are at risk of relapse, seeking help from a healthcare provider or mental health professional can be beneficial. They can provide support and guidance to help you overcome challenges and stay on track.

- Practice self-care: Taking care of yourself is important for maintaining progress and preventing relapse. This can include getting enough sleep, exercising regularly, and taking time for activities that bring you joy and relaxation.

- Manage stress: Stress can be a major barrier to maintaining progress and preventing relapse. Consider incorporating stress management techniques, such as deep breathing, progressive muscle relaxation, and meditation, into your routine.

- Be flexible: It is important to be flexible and adapt to changes in your schedule or circumstances. If you are unable to follow your insulin resistance diet plan as planned, don't be too hard on yourself. Instead, try to make healthy choices and get back on track as soon as possible.

- Have a plan for setbacks: Setbacks are a normal part of the process and are not a reason to give up on your health goals. If you experience a setback, try to identify the cause and come up with a plan to prevent it from happening again in the future.

By following these strategies and being consistent with your insulin resistance diet plan, you can effectively maintain progress and prevent relapse. Remember to work with a healthcare provider and a registered dietitian to develop an eating plan that is right for you and meets your individual needs and goals. It is also important to be kind to yourself and remember that progress takes time. Don't be too hard on yourself if you experience setbacks or challenges along the way. By being patient and persistent, you can successfully manage insulin resistance and improve your overall health.

In addition to the strategies listed above, it can also be helpful to have a support system in place to help you stay on track. This can include friends and family, a healthcare provider, a registered dietitian, or a support group. Having a support system can provide motivation, accountability, and encouragement to help you stay committed to your health goals.

Another important aspect of maintaining progress and preventing relapse is finding ways to incorporate your insulin resistance diet plan into your daily routine. This may involve making small changes to your meals, such as choosing whole grains instead of refined grains, or adding more vegetables to your meals. It may also involve finding ways to incorporate physical activity into your day, such as going for a walk after dinner or taking a yoga class. By finding ways to make healthy habits a part of your routine, you can more easily maintain progress and prevent relapse.

In conclusion, maintaining progress and preventing relapse are important considerations when following an insulin resistance diet plan. By setting specific, achievable goals, creating a supportive environment, practicing self-care, managing stress, and having a plan for setbacks, you can effectively maintain progress and prevent relapse. Remember to work with a healthcare provider and a registered dietitian to develop an eating plan that is right for you and meets your individual needs and goals.

## Incorporating healthy habits into your daily routine

Incorporating healthy habits into your daily routine is an important step in managing insulin resistance and improving overall health. Here are some tips for incorporating healthy habits into your daily routine:

- Get enough sleep: Getting enough sleep is important for both physical and mental health. Aim for 7-9 hours of sleep per night and create a consistent sleep routine to help improve sleep quality.

- Exercise regularly: Exercise is a great way to reduce stress and improve insulin sensitivity. Try to engage in 30 minutes of moderate exercise, like brisk walking or cycling, on a daily basis.

- Eat a balanced diet: A balanced diet that includes a variety of low-glycemic foods, such as fruits and vegetables, whole grains, legumes, nuts and seeds, and lean protein sources, can help keep blood sugar levels stable and reduce the risk of insulin resistance.

- Manage stress: Stress can impact insulin sensitivity and blood sugar control. Practice relaxation techniques, such as deep breathing and meditation, to help manage stress and improve insulin sensitivity.

- Stay hydrated: Drinking an adequate amount of water is crucial for maintaining good health. Try to consume at least 8 cups of water daily to ensure proper hydration.

- Practice self-care: Taking care of yourself is important for both physical and mental health. Make time for activities that you enjoy and prioritize self-care to help you stay motivated and on track with your health goals.

By incorporating these healthy habits into your daily routine, you can effectively manage insulin resistance and improve your overall health. Remember to work with a healthcare provider and a registered dietitian to develop an individualized plan that meets

your specific needs and goals.

# Managing insulin resistance during special occasions and eating out

Managing insulin resistance during special occasions and eating out can be a challenge, but it is possible to enjoy yourself while still following a healthy eating plan. Here are some tips for managing insulin resistance during special occasions and eating out:

- Plan ahead: If you know you will be eating out or attending a special occasion, plan ahead by looking at the menu in advance or bringing your own food if possible. This can help you make informed choices and stick to your insulin resistance diet plan.

- Make healthy choices: When eating out, choose dishes that are lower in calories and fat and focus on whole, unprocessed foods. Look for dishes that are high in protein and fiber and low on the glycemic index.

- Be mindful of portion sizes: It can be easy to eat more than you intended when eating out, especially if the portions are larger than usual. Be mindful of portion sizes and consider sharing a dish or taking some food home for leftovers.

- Don't be afraid to make special requests: Most restaurants are willing to accommodate special requests, such as leaving out certain ingredients or substituting certain items. Don't be afraid to speak up and ask for what you need to follow your insulin resistance diet plan.

- Practice moderation: It is okay to indulge in treats or foods that may not be part of your usual insulin-resistance diet plan, but be sure to practice moderation. Enjoy a small portion of your favorite treat and balance it out with healthy choices the rest of the time.

- Stay active: Incorporating physical activity into your routine can help offset the effects of any indulgences and can also help reduce stress.

By following these tips and being mindful of your food choices, you can manage insulin resistance during special occasions and eating out. Remember to work with a healthcare provider and a registered dietitian to develop an eating plan that is right for you and meets your individual needs and goals.

# Chapter 6

## Working with Your Healthcare Team

Working with a healthcare team is an important aspect of managing insulin resistance. Your healthcare team may include a primary care provider, a specialist such as an endocrinologist or a registered dietitian, and other healthcare professionals, such as a pharmacist or physical therapist. It is important to communicate with your healthcare team regularly and seek their guidance and support to help manage insulin resistance effectively.

In this chapter, we will discuss the importance of working with a healthcare team, tips for communicating with your healthcare provider, and how medication and insulin therapy can be used to manage insulin resistance. By working closely with your healthcare team, you can take control of your health and effectively manage insulin resistance.

## The importance of working with a healthcare team

Working with a healthcare team is an important aspect of managing insulin resistance and maintaining overall health. A healthcare team may include a primary care provider, a specialist such as an endocrinologist, and other healthcare professionals, such as a pharmacist or physical therapist. Each member of the team plays a specific role in your healthcare and works together to help you manage your condition effectively. Here are some reasons why it is important to work with a healthcare team:

- Comprehensive care: A healthcare team can provide comprehensive care that addresses all aspects of your health, including physical, mental, and emotional well-being. By working with a team of professionals, you can receive a range of services and support that are tailored to your individual needs and goals.

- Expertise and knowledge: Healthcare professionals are experts in their field and can provide guidance and support based on the latest research and evidence. They can help you understand your condition and develop a plan that is right for you.

- Coordinated care: A healthcare team can help coordinate your care and ensure that all aspects of your health are being addressed. For example, if you have insulin resistance and are also dealing with high blood pressure, your healthcare team can work together to develop a plan that addresses both conditions.

- Ongoing support: A healthcare team can provide ongoing support and guidance to help you manage your condition effectively. They can help you make necessary lifestyle changes, such as adopting a low-glycemic diet and getting regular physical activity and can also provide support and encouragement to help you stick to your plan.

- Improved outcomes: Working with a healthcare team has been shown to improve health outcomes. By receiving comprehensive and coordinated care, you can effectively manage insulin resistance and improve your overall health.

It is important to communicate with your healthcare team regularly and seek their guidance and support to help manage insulin resistance effectively. Remember to ask questions and express any concerns you may have, as your healthcare team is there to help you. You can also bring a family member or friend to your appointments to help support you and advocate for your health.

It is also important to follow the advice and treatment plan recommended by your healthcare team. This may include taking medications as prescribed, following a specific diet and exercise plan, and attending regular appointments. By working closely with your healthcare team and following their recommendations, you can take control of your health and effectively manage insulin resistance.

Remember, managing insulin resistance is a lifelong process, and it is important to be consistent and make changes to your diet and lifestyle that are sustainable. Working with a healthcare team can provide the support and guidance you need to make lasting changes and improve your overall health.

# Tips for communicating with your healthcare provider

Effective communication with your healthcare provider is an important aspect of managing insulin resistance and overall health. Here are some tips for communicating with your healthcare provider:

- Prepare for your appointment: Before your appointment, make a list of questions or concerns you want to discuss with your healthcare provider. Consider bringing a family member or friend with you to the appointment for additional support.

- Be open and honest: Share any relevant information with your healthcare provider, including your symptoms, medical history, and lifestyle habits. It is important to be honest, and open so that your healthcare provider can develop an accurate understanding of your health and provide the best care possible.

- Ask questions: Don't be afraid to ask questions during your appointment. It is important to understand your health and treatment options, and your healthcare provider is there to help you.

- Take notes: Consider bringing a notepad or using your phone to take notes during your appointment. This can help you remember what was discussed and any recommendations made by your healthcare provider.

- Follow-up: If you have any additional questions or concerns after your appointment, don't hesitate to follow up with your healthcare provider. They are there to support you and help you manage your health.

By following these tips and being an active participant in your healthcare, you can effectively communicate with your healthcare provider and work together to manage insulin resistance and improve your overall health. It is important to remember that managing insulin resistance is a team effort, and it is essential to work closely with your healthcare provider to develop a plan that

is right for you.

# Managing insulin resistance with medication and insulin therapy

Medication and insulin therapy can be an effective way to manage insulin resistance and improve blood sugar control. It is important to work with a healthcare provider to determine the best treatment plan for your specific needs and goals. Here is an overview of how medication and insulin therapy can be used to manage insulin resistance:

- Medications for insulin resistance: There are several medications that can be used to manage insulin resistance, including metformin and thiazolidinediones. Metformin is a common first-line treatment for insulin resistance and is usually taken in pill form. Thiazolidinediones, also known as TZDs, are another type of medication that can be used to treat insulin resistance. These medications work by increasing the sensitivity of cells to insulin, which can help improve blood sugar control.

- Insulin therapy: Insulin therapy involves taking insulin injections or using an insulin pump to deliver insulin to the body. Insulin is a hormone that is produced by the pancreas and is necessary for the body to use glucose for energy. People with insulin resistance may not produce enough insulin or may not use it effectively, which can lead to high blood sugar levels. Insulin therapy can help manage insulin resistance by providing the body with the insulin it needs to effectively use glucose.

- Combination therapy: It is common for people with insulin resistance to use a combination of medications and insulin therapy to manage their condition. This may involve taking a combination of medications, such as metformin and a TZD, and using insulin injections or an insulin pump. It is important to work with a healthcare provider to determine the best treatment plan for your specific needs and goals.

It is important to note that medication and insulin therapy are not a cure for insulin resistance, and they should be used in conjunction with lifestyle changes, such as following a low-glycemic diet and getting regular physical activity, to effectively manage the condition. It is also important to work closely with a healthcare provider and follow their instructions and recommendations to ensure the safe and effective use of medication and insulin therapy.

In addition to medication and insulin therapy, there are other treatments that may be recommended for managing insulin resistance. These may include:

- Incretin-based therapies: Incretin-based therapies, such as GLP-1 receptor agonists and DPP-4 inhibitors, can be used to manage insulin resistance and improve blood sugar control. These medications work by increasing the production of insulin and decreasing the production of glucagon, which can help improve blood sugar control.

- Bariatric surgery: In severe cases of insulin resistance, bariatric surgery may be recommended. This type of surgery involves making changes to the digestive system to help people lose weight and improve insulin sensitivity.

It is important to work with a healthcare provider to determine the best treatment plan for managing insulin resistance. By following the recommended treatment plan and making necessary lifestyle changes, you can effectively manage insulin resistance and improve your overall health.

# Chapter 7

## Delicious, Low-Glycemic Recipes

In this chapter, you will find a variety of tasty and healthy recipes that are perfect for anyone looking to manage insulin resistance and improve blood sugar control. The recipes in this chapter are all low on the glycemic index, which means they are absorbed more slowly by the body and can help keep blood sugar levels stable. You will find breakfast, lunch, dinner, and snack recipes to help you fuel your body throughout the day. Whether you are looking for something quick and easy or a more elaborate meal, this chapter has something for everyone. These recipes are not only delicious, but they are also healthy and can help you take control of your health and manage insulin resistance effectively.

# Breakfast recipes to kick-start your day

## Overnight oats with berries and nuts

**Description:** This easy and convenient breakfast option is made by soaking oats in liquid overnight, allowing them to soften and absorb the flavors of the other ingredients. This recipe adds a burst of sweetness from berries and a crunch from nuts for a tasty and satisfying breakfast.

**Preparation time:** 5 minutes (plus at least 8 hours for soaking)

**Cook time:** 0 minutes

**Ingredients:**

- 1 cup rolled oats
- 1 cup milk or yogurt
- 1/2 cup chopped berries
- 1/4 cup chopped nuts or seeds

**Preparation:**

- In a medium bowl or jar, combine the oats, milk or yogurt, and berries. Stir until the oats are evenly coated in the liquid. Cover the bowl or jar with a lid or plastic wrap and refrigerate for at least 8 hours or overnight.

- In the morning, stir in the chopped nuts or seeds and divide the oats into bowls. Serve chilled or at room temperature.

# Avocado toast with egg and tomato

**Description:** This simple yet flavorful breakfast combines the creamy goodness of avocado with the protein of an egg and the freshness of a tomato on top of toasted bread. It's a quick and easy way to fuel your body and start your day off right.

**Preparation time:** 5 minutes

**Cook time:** 5 minutes

**Ingredients:**

- 1 slice bread
- 1/2 avocado
- 1 egg
- 1 tomato, sliced
- Salt and pepper to taste

**Preparation:**

- Toast the bread to your desired level of doneness.

- Spread the avocado evenly over the toast.

- Heat a small skillet over medium heat. Crack the egg into the skillet and cook until the white is set and the yolk is cooked to your desired level of doneness.

- Top the avocado toast with the sliced tomato and the cooked egg. Season with salt and pepper to taste. Serve immediately.

# Whole grain waffles with fruit and yogurt

**Description:** These whole-grain waffles are a tasty and healthier alternative to traditional waffles, and they are topped with a delicious mix of fruit and yogurt for a satisfying breakfast.

**Preparation time:** 5 minutes

**Cook time:** 15 minutes

**Ingredients:**

- 1 cup whole wheat flour

- 1 cup all-purpose flour

- 1 tsp baking powder

- 1 cup milk

- 1 egg

- 1 tbsp vegetable oil

- 1 cup fruit (such as berries, sliced apples, or chopped bananas)

- 1 cup plain yogurt

**Preparation:**

- In a medium bowl, mix together the whole wheat flour, all-purpose flour, and baking powder.

- In a separate bowl, whisk together the milk, egg, and vegetable oil.

- Pour the wet ingredients into the dry ingredients and mix until just combined.

- Preheat a waffle iron and spray with non-stick cooking spray. Pour the batter into the waffle iron and cook until the waffles are golden brown and crisp.

- Top the waffles with the fruit and yogurt, and serve.

# Scrambled eggs with spinach and tomatoes

**Description:** This simple and satisfying breakfast combines scrambled eggs with flavorful and nutritious spinach and tomatoes for a tasty and wholesome meal.

**Preparation time:** 5 minutes

**Cook time:** 10 minutes

**Ingredients:**

- 2 eggs

- 1 cup spinach, chopped

- 1/2 cup diced tomatoes

- 1 tsp butter

- Salt and pepper, to taste

**Preparation:**

- In a small skillet, melt the butter over medium heat.

- Whisk together the eggs in a small bowl and pour them into the skillet.

- Stir in the chopped spinach and diced tomatoes.

- Cook the eggs, stirring occasionally until they are fully cooked and scrambled.

- Season with salt and pepper to taste, and serve.

# Turkey and Cheese Omelette

**Description:** This protein-packed omelette is filled with flavorful turkey and melted cheese, making it a perfect breakfast option for those on the go.

**Preparation time:** 5 minutes

**Cook time:** 5 minutes

**Ingredients:**

- 2 large eggs
- 1/4 cup diced cooked turkey
- 1/4 cup shredded cheese
- 1 tablespoon butter

**Preparation:**

- Heat a small non-stick frying pan over medium heat.
- Whisk together the eggs in a small bowl.
- Melt the butter in the frying pan and pour in the eggs.

- Stir in the diced turkey and sprinkle the cheese over the
  top.

- Cook the omelette until the edges start to turn golden
  brown, about 3-4 minutes.

- Flip the omelette and cook for an additional 1-2 minutes
  until the cheese is melted and the omelette is cooked
  through.

- Slide the omelette out of the pan and onto a plate. Enjoy!

# Greek Yogurt with Granola and Fruit

**Description:** This refreshing breakfast bowl is filled with creamy Greek yogurt, crunchy granola, and sweet fruit, making it a delicious and healthy way to start the day.

**Preparation time:** 5 minutes

**Cook time:** 0 minutes

**Ingredients:**

- 1 cup Greek yogurt
- 1/2 cup granola
- 1 cup chopped fruit (such as berries, apples, or bananas)

**Preparation:**

- In a medium bowl, combine the Greek yogurt and granola.
- Stir in the chopped fruit.
- Divide the mixture into bowls and serve. Enjoy!

# Quiche with Vegetables and Whole Grain Crust

**Description:** This savory quiche is filled with a variety of vegetables and baked in a whole-grain crust, making it a healthy and satisfying meal option.

**Preparation time:** 15 minutes

**Cook time:** 45 minutes

**Ingredients:**

- 1 cup whole wheat flour

- 1/2 cup cold butter, diced

- 1/4 cup ice water

- 1 cup diced vegetables (such as bell peppers, onions, and spinach)

- 1 cup shredded cheese

- 4 eggs

- 1 cup milk

- 1 tsp salt

- 1/2 tsp pepper

**Preparation:**

- To make the crust, combine the flour and butter in a food processor and pulse until the mixture resembles coarse sand. Add the ice water and pulse until the dough comes together. Roll the dough out into a 12-inch circle and transfer to a 9-inch pie dish.

- In a separate bowl, whisk together the eggs, milk, salt, and pepper. Stir in the diced vegetables and shredded cheese. Pour the mixture into the pie dish.

- Bake the quiche at 350°F for 45 minutes, or until the crust is golden brown and the filling is set. Allow to cool for a few minutes before slicing and serving.

# Whole Grain Pancake with Peanut Butter and Banana

**Description:** These fluffy whole grain pancakes are topped with creamy peanut butter and sliced bananas for a delicious and nourishing breakfast option.

**Preparation time:** 10 minutes

**Cook time:** 15 minutes

**Ingredients:**

- 1 cup whole wheat flour

- 1 tsp baking powder

- 1/2 tsp salt

- 1 cup milk

- 1 egg

- 1 tbsp vegetable oil

- 1/4 cup peanut butter

- 1 banana, sliced

**Preparation:**

- In a medium bowl, whisk together the flour, baking powder, and salt. In a separate bowl, beat together the milk, egg, and oil. Add the wet ingredients to the dry ingredients and stir until just combined.

- Heat a griddle or large nonstick skillet over medium heat. Drop spoonfuls of the batter onto the griddle and cook until bubbles form on the surface and the edges are set. Flip and cook until the other side is golden brown.

- Repeat the process until all the batter is used up. Top the pancakes with peanut butter and sliced bananas before serving.

# Breakfast burrito with beans, egg, and avocado

**Description:** This flavorful breakfast burrito is filled with protein-rich beans, a hearty egg, and creamy avocado, making it a satisfying and nourishing way to start the day.

**Preparation time:** 10 minutes

**Cook time:** 10 minutes

**Ingredients:**

- 1 small can black beans, rinsed and drained
- 1 egg
- 1/2 avocado, diced
- 1 small tortilla
- Optional toppings: salsa, cheese, cilantro, lime wedges

**Preparation:**

- In a small saucepan, heat the black beans over medium heat until heated through.

- In a separate small pan, fry the egg over medium heat until the whites are set and the yolk is cooked to your desired doneness.

- Assemble the burrito by laying the tortilla flat and adding the heated beans, fried egg, and diced avocado. Top with any desired toppings and roll the tortilla into a burrito shape. Serve immediately.

# Smoothie bowl with spinach, banana, and berries

**Description:** This refreshing smoothie bowl is packed with nutrients from the spinach, banana, and berries, and it makes for a delicious and healthy breakfast or snack.

**Preparation time:** 5 minutes

**Cook time:** 0 minutes

**Ingredients:**

- 1 cup frozen berries (such as strawberries, blueberries, or raspberries)
- 1 banana
- 1 cup fresh spinach
- 1 cup almond milk or water
- Optional toppings: granola, nuts, seeds, coconut flakes, fresh fruit

**Preparation:**

- Combine the frozen berries, banana, spinach, and almond milk or water in a blender and blend until smooth.

- Pour the smoothie into a bowl and top with any desired toppings. Serve immediately.

# Whole grain toast with avocado and hard-boiled egg

**Description:** This healthy and satisfying breakfast combines creamy avocado and protein-rich eggs with whole grain toast for a balanced and delicious start to the day.

**Preparation time:** 5 minutes

**Cook time:** 5 minutes

**Ingredients:**

- 2 slices whole grain bread

- 1 avocado, mashed

- 1 hard-boiled egg, sliced

- Salt and pepper, to taste

**Preparation:**

- Toast the bread to your desired level of doneness.

- Spread the mashed avocado on top of the toast.

- Top with sliced hard-boiled egg and sprinkle with salt and

  pepper.

- Serve immediately.

# Omelette with vegetables and feta cheese

**Description:** This omelette is a great way to get in your daily serving of vegetables and protein, all while enjoying a delicious and filling breakfast.

**Preparation time:** 10 minutes

**Cook time:** 10 minutes

**Ingredients:**

- 2 eggs

- 1/2 cup mixed vegetables (such as bell peppers, onions, and mushrooms)

- 1/4 cup feta cheese, crumbled

- Salt and pepper, to taste

- 1 tablespoon butter or oil

**Preparation:**

- Beat the eggs in a small bowl and set aside.

- Heat the butter or oil in a small skillet over medium heat.

- Add the mixed vegetables and cook until they are tender, about 5 minutes.

- Pour the beaten eggs over the vegetables and sprinkle with feta cheese.

- Cook until the eggs are set and the cheese is melted, about 5 minutes.

- Season with salt and pepper, to taste.

- Serve immediately.

# Whole grain muffins with nuts and fruit

**Description:** These wholesome muffins are packed with nutrients and flavor, thanks to the combination of whole grain flour, nuts, and fruit. They make a great snack or breakfast option.

**Preparation time:** 10 minutes

**Cook time:** 20 minutes

**Ingredients:**

- 1 cup whole grain flour
- 1 teaspoon baking powder
- 1/4 teaspoon salt
- 1 egg
- 1/4 cup oil
- 1/4 cup milk
- 1/4 cup chopped nuts (such as almonds or walnuts)
- 1/4 cup chopped fruit (such as berries or diced apples)

**Preparation:**

- Preheat the oven to 350°F. Line a muffin tin with paper liners.

- In a medium bowl, mix together the flour, baking powder, and salt.

- In a separate bowl, beat the egg and then stir in the oil and milk.

- Pour the wet ingredients into the dry ingredients and stir just until combined.

- Fold in the nuts and fruit.

- Divide the batter evenly among the muffin cups.

- Bake for 18-20 minutes, or until a toothpick inserted into the center of a muffin comes out clean.

# Whole grain cereal with milk and fruit

**Description:** This simple but nutritious breakfast option combines whole grain cereal with milk and fruit for a balanced meal that is rich in protein, fiber, and nutrients.

**Preparation time:** 2 minutes

**Cook time:** 0 minutes

**Ingredients:**

- 1 cup whole grain cereal (such as oats, barley, or quinoa)
- 1 cup milk (cow's milk, almond milk, or soy milk)
- 1/2 cup chopped fruit (such as berries, apples, or bananas)

**Preparation:**

- Pour the cereal into a bowl.
- Add the milk and stir to combine.
- Top with the chopped fruit and serve.

# Whole grain toast with peanut butter and honey

**Description:** This simple and satisfying breakfast combines the nutritious goodness of whole grains with the protein-rich goodness of peanut butter and the natural sweetness of honey.

**Preparation time:** 5 minutes

**Cook time:** 5 minutes

**Ingredients:**

- 2 slices of whole grain bread

- 2 tablespoons peanut butter

- 1 tablespoon honey

**Preparation:**

- Toast the bread in a toaster or on a stovetop griddle until it is lightly browned and crisp.

- Spread the peanut butter evenly over the toast, then drizzle the honey over the top.

- Serve immediately.

# Whole grain crepes with berries and yogurt

**Description:** This delicious and light breakfast combines the wholesome goodness of whole grains with the antioxidant-rich goodness of berries and the protein-rich goodness of yogurt.

**Preparation time:** 10 minutes

**Cook time:** 20 minutes

**Ingredients:**

- 1 cup whole grain flour
- 2 eggs
- 1 cup milk
- 1/2 cup chopped berries (such as strawberries, raspberries, or blueberries)
- 1 cup plain yogurt

**Preparation:**

- In a blender or food processor, combine the flour, eggs, and milk and blend until smooth.

- Heat a large nonstick skillet over medium heat and lightly coat with cooking spray.

- Pour about 1/4 cup of the crepe batter into the skillet and swirl to coat the bottom of the skillet evenly.

- Cook the crepe for about 1-2 minutes, or until the edges start to curl and the bottom is lightly browned.

- Flip the crepe and cook for another minute, or until the other side is lightly browned.

- Repeat with the remaining batter to make 4-6 crepes.

- Divide the crepes among plates, top with the chopped berries and yogurt, and serve.

# Egg and Vegetable Scramble

**Description:** This protein-packed breakfast is filled with flavorful vegetables and eggs, making it a healthy and satisfying way to start the day.

**Preparation time:** 10 minutes

**Cook time:** 10 minutes

**Ingredients:**

- 2 eggs

- 1/2 cup diced vegetables (such as bell peppers, onions, and mushrooms)

- 1 tablespoon olive oil

- Salt and pepper, to taste

**Preparation:**

- Heat the olive oil in a small skillet over medium heat.

- Add the diced vegetables and cook for 5-7 minutes, until they are tender.

- Crack the eggs into the skillet and stir gently to combine with the vegetables.

- Cook for an additional 2-3 minutes, until the eggs are fully cooked.

- Season with salt and pepper, to taste.

- Serve hot.

# Whole Grain Waffles with Eggs and Bacon

**Description:** This savory breakfast combines crispy bacon and fluffy waffles with a delicious fried egg on top, creating a satisfying and tasty meal.

**Preparation time:** 10 minutes

**Cook time:** 20 minutes

**Ingredients:**

- 1 cup whole grain waffle mix

- 1 egg

- 1/2 cup water

- 1/4 cup diced bacon

- 1 egg

**Preparation:**

- Mix the waffle mix, egg, and water in a medium bowl until well combined.

- Preheat a waffle iron and spray with cooking spray.

- Pour the waffle batter into the iron and cook according to the manufacturer's instructions.

- While the waffle is cooking, heat a small skillet over medium heat and add the diced bacon.

- Cook the bacon for 5-7 minutes, until crispy.

- Crack the egg into the skillet and fry until the white is set and the yolk is desired doneness.

- Once the waffle is finished cooking, place it on a plate and top with the fried egg and crispy bacon. Serve hot.

# Whole grain toast with hummus and vegetables

**Description:** This savory and satisfying breakfast provides a balance of whole grains, protein, and vegetables, and it can be a delicious and nourishing way to start the day.

**Preparation time:** 5 minutes

**Cook time:** 0 minutes

**Ingredients:**

- 2 slices of whole grain bread

- 1/4 cup hummus

- 1/2 cup chopped vegetables (such as bell peppers, cucumbers, or tomatoes)

**Preparation:**

- Toast the bread until it is crispy and golden brown.

- Spread the hummus on the toast and top with the chopped vegetables.

- Slice the toast into wedges and serve.

# Breakfast smoothie with protein powder and berries

**Description:** This refreshing and satisfying breakfast smoothie provides a balance of protein, carbohydrates, and healthy fats, and it can be a delicious and nourishing way to start the day.

**Preparation time:** 5 minutes

**Cook time:** 0 minutes

**Ingredients:**

- 1 cup milk or milk alternative

- 1 scoop protein powder

- 1 cup frozen berries

- 1/2 banana

- 1 tsp honey (optional)

**Preparation:**

- Place all ingredients in a blender and blend until smooth.

- Pour the smoothie into a glass and serve.

# Lunch recipes to fuel you through the afternoon

## Quinoa and Black Bean Salad with Avocado Dressing

**Description:** This healthy and flavorful salad combines the nutrients of quinoa and black beans with the creamy goodness of avocado dressing. It's perfect for a light lunch or dinner.

**Preparation time:** 15 minutes

**Cook time:** 20 minutes

**Ingredients:**

- 1 cup quinoa
- 2 cups water
- 1 cup cooked black beans
- 1 cup diced vegetables (such as bell peppers, tomatoes, and onions)
- 1 avocado
- 1/4 cup olive oil
- 1/4 cup lemon juice
- Salt and pepper to taste

**Preparation:**

- Bring the water to a boil in a small saucepan over medium-high heat.
- Stir in the quinoa and reduce the heat to medium-low.
- Cook the quinoa for about 15-20 minutes, or until it is fluffy and the water is absorbed.
- Meanwhile, mash the avocado in a small bowl and stir in the olive oil, lemon juice, salt, and pepper.
- In a large bowl, combine the cooked quinoa, black beans, and diced vegetables.
- Drizzle the avocado dressing over the top and toss to coat. Serve chilled or at room temperature.

# Grilled Chicken and Vegetable Skewers with a Side of Quinoa

**Description:** This simple and satisfying meal features flavorful grilled chicken and vegetables paired with the nutty goodness of quinoa.

**Preparation time:** 15 minutes

**Cook time:** 20 minutes

**Ingredients:**

- 1 cup quinoa
- 2 cups water
- 1 pound chicken breast, cut into 1-inch pieces
- 1 cup diced vegetables (such as bell peppers, onions, and cherry tomatoes)
- 1/4 cup olive oil
- 1/4 cup lemon juice
- Salt and pepper to taste

**Preparation:**

- Soak wooden skewers in water for at least 15 minutes to prevent them from burning on the grill.

- Preheat the grill to medium-high heat.

- In a small saucepan, bring the water to a boil over medium-high heat.

- Stir in the quinoa and reduce the heat to medium-low.

- Cook the quinoa for about 15-20 minutes, or until it is fluffy and the water is absorbed.

- Meanwhile, thread the chicken and vegetables onto the skewers.

- Brush the skewers with the olive oil and sprinkle with salt and pepper.

- Grill the skewers for about 8-10 minutes, turning occasionally, until the chicken is cooked through and the vegetables are tender.

- Serve the skewers with the quinoa on the side.

# Whole grain turkey and cheese wrap with lettuce, tomato, and hummus

**Description:** This healthy and delicious wrap is filled with protein-rich turkey and cheese, and topped with refreshing lettuce, tomato, and creamy hummus. It's a quick and easy meal that's perfect for on-the-go lunches or a light dinner.

**Preparation time:** 10 minutes

**Cook time:** 0 minutes

**Ingredients:**

- 1 whole grain tortilla
- 1/4 cup sliced turkey
- 1 slice cheese
- 1 leaf lettuce
- 1 slice tomato
- 2 tablespoons hummus

**Preparation:**

- Lay the tortilla out on a flat surface.

- Arrange the turkey and cheese slices on one side of the tortilla.

- Top with the lettuce, tomato, and hummus.

- Fold the tortilla over the fillings and press gently to seal.

- Slice the wrap in half and serve.

# Grilled salmon with roasted vegetables and brown rice

**Description:** This hearty and flavorful meal features succulent grilled salmon, paired with roasted vegetables and nutty brown rice. It's a complete and well-balanced dinner that's sure to satisfy.

**Preparation time:** 10 minutes

**Cook time:** 20 minutes

**Ingredients:**

- 1 salmon fillet
- 1 cup mixed vegetables (such as bell peppers, onions, and zucchini)
- 1/2 cup brown rice
- 1 tablespoon olive oil
- 1 teaspoon garlic powder
- 1 teaspoon dried herbs (such as oregano or basil)

**Preparation:**

- Preheat the oven to 400 degrees F.

- Toss the vegetables in a bowl with the olive oil, garlic powder, and herbs.

- Spread the vegetables on a baking sheet and roast for 15-20 minutes, until tender and caramelized.

- Meanwhile, heat a grill pan over medium-high heat.

- Spray the pan with cooking spray and place the salmon fillet on it.

- Grill the salmon for 5-7 minutes on each side, until it is cooked through and flakes easily.

- Cook the brown rice according to package instructions.

- Serve the salmon, vegetables, and rice in bowls or on plates.

# Black bean and corn salad with grilled chicken

**Description:** This refreshing and flavorful salad is packed with protein, fiber, and nutrients from the black beans, corn, and grilled chicken. It's a healthy and satisfying meal that can be enjoyed on its own or as a side dish.

**Preparation time:** 15 minutes

**Cook time:** 15 minutes

**Ingredients:**

- 1 can black beans, drained and rinsed
- 1 cup corn kernels (fresh or frozen)
- 1 bell pepper, diced
- 1 small red onion, diced
- 1/4 cup chopped cilantro
- 1/4 cup olive oil
- 1 tbsp red wine vinegar
- 1 tsp chili powder

- 1/2 tsp ground cumin

- 1/2 tsp salt

- 1 lb grilled chicken, sliced

**Preparation:**

- In a medium bowl, mix together the black beans, corn, bell pepper, red onion, and cilantro.

- In a small bowl, whisk together the olive oil, red wine vinegar, chili powder, cumin, and salt.

- Pour the dressing over the bean and corn mixture and toss to coat.

- Arrange the grilled chicken slices on top of the salad and serve.

# Whole grain spaghetti with turkey meatballs and steamed broccoli

**Description:** This hearty and nutritious meal combines whole grain spaghetti, lean turkey meatballs, and steamed broccoli for a balance of carbohydrates, protein, and vegetables. It's a simple and delicious way to get your daily serving of nutrients.

**Preparation time:** 15 minutes

**Cook time:** 25 minutes

**Ingredients:**

- 1 lb whole grain spaghetti

- 1 lb ground turkey

- 1/2 cup bread crumbs

- 1 egg, beaten

- 1/4 cup grated parmesan cheese

- 1 tsp Italian seasoning

- 1/2 tsp salt

- 1/4 tsp black pepper

- 1 cup broccoli florets

- 1 tbsp olive oil

- 1/4 cup tomato sauce

**Preparation:**

- Bring a large pot of salted water to a boil and cook the spaghetti according to package instructions.

- Meanwhile, in a medium bowl, mix together the ground turkey, bread crumbs, egg, parmesan cheese, Italian seasoning, salt, and pepper. Form the mixture into small meatballs.

- Heat the olive oil in a large skillet over medium-high heat.

- Add the meatballs and cook for about 5-7 minutes, until they are browned on all sides.

- Add the tomato sauce and simmer for an additional 5 minutes.

- In a small saucepan, bring a small amount of water to a boil and steam the broccoli florets for about 3-5 minutes, until they are tender.

- Drain the spaghetti and divide it into bowls. Top each serving with the meatballs, tomato sauce, and steamed broccoli. Serve hot.

# Turkey and avocado lettuce cups with cherry tomatoes and cucumbers

**Description:** These refreshing and satisfying lettuce cups are filled with protein-rich turkey, creamy avocado, and crunchy cherry tomatoes and cucumbers. A healthy and flavorful lunch or dinner option.

**Preparation time:** 10 minutes

**Cook time:** 5 minutes

**Ingredients:**

- 4 lettuce leaves

- 4 ounces sliced turkey

- 1 avocado, sliced

- 1/2 cup cherry tomatoes, halved

- 1/2 cup cucumber, sliced

**Preparation:**

- Heat a grill pan over medium-high heat. Grill the turkey slices for about 2-3 minutes per side, until cooked through.

- Divide the grilled turkey, avocado slices, cherry tomatoes, and cucumber slices among the lettuce leaves.

- Serve the lettuce cups immediately.

# Grilled chicken and vegetable stir-fry with brown rice

**Description:** This flavorful and healthy stir-fry combines tender grilled chicken with a variety of colorful and nutritious vegetables, served over a bed of nutty and whole grain brown rice.

**Preparation time:** 15 minutes

**Cook time:** 20 minutes

**Ingredients:**

- 1 pound chicken breasts, sliced into thin strips
- 1 cup brown rice
- 2 cups water
- 1 tablespoon vegetable oil
- 1 red bell pepper, sliced
- 1 yellow bell pepper, sliced
- 1 cup sliced mushrooms
- 1 cup chopped broccoli
- 1 cup chopped carrots

- 2 cloves garlic, minced

- 1 tablespoon soy sauce

- 1 tablespoon hoisin sauce

**Preparation:**

- Cook the brown rice according to package instructions, using 2 cups of water.

- Heat the vegetable oil in a large wok or skillet over high heat.

- Add the chicken strips and cook for about 4-5 minutes, until cooked through.

- Remove the chicken from the wok and set aside.

- Add the bell peppers, mushrooms, broccoli, and carrots to the wok and cook for about 5-7 minutes, until the vegetables are tender.

- Add the garlic and cook for another minute.

- Stir in the soy sauce and hoisin sauce.

- Return the cooked chicken to the wok and stir to combine
  with the vegetables.

- Serve the chicken and vegetable stir-fry over the cooked
  brown rice.

# Whole grain pita with hummus, tomato, cucumber, and lettuce

**Description:** This flavorful and healthy sandwich is packed with protein, fiber, and nutrients from the whole grain pita, hummus, and vegetables. It's a quick and easy meal that can be enjoyed for lunch or dinner.

**Preparation time**: 5 minutes

**Cook time:** 0 minutes

**Ingredients:**

- 1 whole grain pita bread
- 1/4 cup hummus
- 1 small tomato, sliced
- 1/2 small cucumber, sliced
- 1/2 cup lettuce, chopped

**Preparation:**

- Slice the pita bread in half to create two pockets.

- Spread the hummus evenly inside each pocket.

- Arrange the tomato, cucumber, and lettuce slices inside the pockets.

- Close the pockets and cut each one in half. Serve immediately.

# Grilled chicken and vegetable salad with a side of whole grain bread

**Description:** This hearty and flavorful meal combines the protein and nutrients of grilled chicken and vegetables with the fiber and complex carbohydrates of whole grain bread. It's a satisfying and healthy option for lunch or dinner.

**Preparation time:** 10 minutes

**Cook time:** 15 minutes

**Ingredients:**

- 1/2 pound boneless, skinless chicken breasts
- 1 cup mixed vegetables (such as bell peppers, zucchini, and onions)
- 1 tablespoon olive oil
- Salt and pepper, to taste
- 1 cup mixed salad greens
- 1/4 cup vinaigrette dressing
- 2 slices whole grain bread

**Preparation:**

- Preheat the grill to medium-high heat.

- Brush the chicken breasts and vegetables with the olive oil and sprinkle with salt and pepper.

- Grill the chicken and vegetables for about 7-8 minutes per side, or until the chicken is cooked through and the vegetables are tender.

- Slice the chicken and vegetables into bite-sized pieces.

- In a large bowl, toss the salad greens with the vinaigrette dressing.

- Divide the salad onto two plates and top with the grilled chicken and vegetables.

- Serve with the whole grain bread on the side.

# Grilled shrimp with quinoa and steamed asparagus

**Description:** This protein-packed and flavorful meal is a great option for a healthy and satisfying dinner. The combination of grilled shrimp, quinoa, and steamed asparagus provides a balance of nutrients and taste.

**Preparation time:** 10 minutes

**Cook time:** 15 minutes

**Ingredients:**

- 1 cup uncooked quinoa
- 2 cups water
- 1 pound shrimp, peeled and deveined
- 1 tablespoon olive oil
- 1 bunch asparagus, trimmed
- Salt and pepper to taste

**Preparation:**

- Rinse the quinoa in a fine mesh strainer and add it to a saucepan with the water. Bring the water to a boil, then reduce the heat to low and simmer for about 15-20 minutes, or until the quinoa is tender and the water has been absorbed.

- Meanwhile, preheat the grill to medium-high heat. Toss the shrimp with the olive oil and season with salt and pepper. Grill the shrimp for about 2-3 minutes per side, or until they are pink and cooked through.

- Steam the asparagus in a steamer basket over boiling water for about 3-5 minutes, or until they are tender but still crisp.

- Divide the quinoa, shrimp, and asparagus onto plates and serve.

# Whole grain pasta with roasted vegetables and grilled chicken

**Description:** This hearty and flavorful pasta dish is a great option for a quick and easy dinner. The combination of whole grain pasta, roasted vegetables, and grilled chicken provides a balance of nutrients and taste.

**Preparation time:** 15 minutes

**Cook time:** 20 minutes

**Ingredients:**

- 8 ounces whole grain pasta
- 1 cup chopped vegetables (such as bell peppers, onions, and zucchini)
- 1 tablespoon olive oil
- 1 pound chicken breasts, sliced into thin strips
- 1 cup marinara sauce
- Salt and pepper to taste

**Preparation:**

- Preheat the oven to 400 degrees F. Line a baking sheet with parchment paper.
- Toss the vegetables with the olive oil and season with salt and pepper. Roast the vegetables in the oven for about 15-20 minutes, or until they are tender and lightly caramelized.
- Meanwhile, bring a pot of salted water to a boil. Add the pasta and cook according to the package instructions.
- Preheat a grill or grill pan to medium-high heat. Grill the chicken for about 3-4 minutes per side, or until it is cooked through.
- Drain the pasta and toss it with the roasted vegetables, grilled chicken, and marinara sauce. Divide the pasta onto plates and serve.

# Grilled tofu and vegetable skewers with a side of brown rice

**Description:** This delicious and healthy meal combines grilled tofu and vegetables with a side of fluffy brown rice. It's a great option for a vegetarian meal or for adding some protein to a side dish.

**Preparation time:** 15 minutes

**Cook time:** 20 minutes

**Ingredients:**

- 1 block firm tofu, cut into 1-inch cubes
- 1 red bell pepper, cut into 1-inch squares
- 1 green bell pepper, cut into 1-inch squares
- 1 small onion, cut into 1-inch squares
- 1 cup brown rice
- 2 cups water
- 1 tsp olive oil
- 1 tsp soy sauce

- 1 tsp garlic powder

- 1 tsp onion powder

**Preparation:**

- Preheat the grill to medium-high heat.
- Thread the tofu and vegetables onto skewers, alternating between each.
- In a small saucepan, bring the water to a boil. Stir in the brown rice and reduce the heat to low. Cover and cook for about 45 minutes, or until the rice is tender.
- Meanwhile, brush the skewers with olive oil and sprinkle with soy sauce, garlic powder, and onion powder. Grill for about 10 minutes, turning once, until the vegetables are tender and the tofu is golden brown.
- Serve the skewers over the brown rice and enjoy.

# Turkey and cheese roll-ups with lettuce and tomato

**Description:** This quick and easy lunch or snack combines sliced turkey and cheese with fresh lettuce and tomato for a tasty and satisfying meal.

**Preparation time:** 5 minutes

**Cook time:** 0 minutes

**Ingredients:**

- 4 slices turkey deli meat
- 2 slices cheese
- 4 lettuce leaves
- 1 tomato, sliced

**Preparation:**

- Lay out the turkey slices on a flat surface. Place a slice of cheese on top of each turkey slice.
- Top with a lettuce leaf and a few tomato slices.

- Roll up the turkey and cheese tightly, securing with toothpicks if needed.

- Slice the roll-ups into bite-sized pieces and serve with additional lettuce and tomato on the side. Enjoy!

# Grilled chicken and vegetable wrap with a side of fruit

**Description:** This flavorful and satisfying meal combines the nutrients of grilled chicken and vegetables with the added bonus of a side of fruit. It's a healthy and convenient option for lunch or dinner.

**Preparation time:** 10 minutes

**Cook time:** 15 minutes

**Ingredients:**

- 1 chicken breast
- 1 whole grain wrap
- 1/2 cup mixed vegetables (such as bell peppers, onions, and zucchini)
- 1 tablespoon olive oil
- 1/2 cup mixed fruit (such as berries, sliced apples, or diced pineapple)

**Preparation:**

- Preheat the grill to medium-high heat.

- Brush the chicken breast and vegetables with olive oil and season with your desired seasonings.

- Grill the chicken and vegetables for about 7-10 minutes on each side, until the chicken is cooked through and the vegetables are tender.

- Slice the chicken and vegetables into thin strips.

- Warm the wrap in the microwave for 30 seconds or on the grill for a few seconds.

- Lay the wrap flat on a clean surface and fill it with the sliced chicken and vegetables. Roll up the wrap tightly and slice it in half on the diagonal.

- Serve the wrap with the side of mixed fruit.

# Whole grain pizza with roasted vegetables and grilled chicken

**Description:** This delicious and healthier version of pizza combines the flavors of grilled chicken and roasted vegetables on a whole grain crust for a satisfying and nutrient-rich meal.

**Preparation time:** 15 minutes

**Cook time:** 20-25 minutes

**Ingredients:**

- 1 whole grain pizza crust
- 1/2 cup tomato sauce
- 1 cup grated mozzarella cheese
- 1/2 cup roasted vegetables (such as bell peppers, onions, and zucchini)
- 1/2 cup diced grilled chicken
- 1/4 cup grated Parmesan cheese

**Preparation:**

- Preheat the oven to 425°F (220°C).

- Place the pizza crust on a large baking sheet.

- Spread the tomato sauce over the crust, leaving a small border around the edges.

- Sprinkle the mozzarella cheese over the tomato sauce.

- Top the cheese with the roasted vegetables and diced chicken.

- Sprinkle the Parmesan cheese over the top.

- Bake the pizza for 20-25 minutes, until the crust is golden brown and the cheese is melted and bubbly.

- Slice the pizza into wedges and serve.

# Grilled salmon with quinoa and steamed broccoli

**Description:** This flavorful and healthy meal combines protein-rich grilled salmon with fiber-packed quinoa and vitamin-rich broccoli for a well-rounded and nutritious dinner option.

**Preparation time:** 10 minutes

**Cook time:** 15 minutes

**Ingredients:**

- 4 oz salmon fillets
- 1 cup quinoa
- 1 cup water
- 1 head of broccoli, cut into florets
- 1 tbsp olive oil
- Salt and pepper to taste

**Preparation:**

- Preheat a grill or grill pan over medium-high heat.
- Season the salmon fillets with salt and pepper.

- Grill the salmon for about 5-7 minutes on each side, or until it is cooked to your desired level of doneness.
- Meanwhile, bring the water to a boil in a small saucepan.
- Stir in the quinoa, reduce the heat to low, and simmer for about 15 minutes, or until the quinoa is cooked and the water is absorbed.
- In a separate pot, bring a small amount of water to a boil.
- Add the broccoli florets and steam for about 5 minutes, or until they are tender but still crisp.
- Serve the grilled salmon on top of the quinoa, with the steamed broccoli on the side.

# Whole grain tortilla with black beans, avocado, and grilled chicken

**Description:** This hearty and flavorful wrap combines protein-rich grilled chicken and black beans with healthy fats from avocado for a satisfying lunch option.

**Preparation time:** 10 minutes

**Cook time:** 15 minutes

**Ingredients:**

- 4 oz grilled chicken, sliced
- 1/2 cup black beans, drained and rinsed
- 1 avocado, mashed
- 2 whole grain tortillas
- 1 tsp olive oil
- Salt and pepper to taste

**Preparation:**

- Preheat a grill or grill pan over medium-high heat.

- Season the chicken with salt and pepper.

- Grill the chicken for about 5-7 minutes on each side, or until it is cooked through.

- Slice the chicken into thin strips.

- Warm the tortillas in a dry skillet over medium heat for about 1-2 minutes on each side, or until they are slightly crispy.

- Spread the mashed avocado over one side of each tortilla.

- Top with the sliced chicken and black beans.

- Fold the tortillas in half and press lightly to seal.

- Brush the tops of the tortillas with a small amount of olive oil.

- Grill the tortillas for about 2-3 minutes on each side, or until they are crispy and browned.

- Slice the tortillas into wedges and serve.

# Grilled chicken and vegetable skewers with a side of quinoa and fruit

**Description:** This flavorful and healthy meal combines grilled chicken and vegetables with a nutritious side of quinoa and fruit. It is a great option for a quick and satisfying dinner.

**Preparation time:** 15 minutes

**Cook time:** 15 minutes

**Ingredients:**

- 1 pound chicken breasts, cut into 1-inch pieces
- 1 bell pepper, cut into 1-inch pieces
- 1 onion, cut into 1-inch pieces
- 1 zucchini, cut into 1-inch pieces
- 1 cup quinoa
- 2 cups water
- 1 cup diced fruit (such as apples, pears, or peaches)
- Skewers

**Preparation:**

- Preheat the grill to medium-high heat.

- Thread the chicken and vegetables onto the skewers.

- Cook the skewers for about 8-10 minutes, turning occasionally, until the chicken is cooked through and the vegetables are tender.

- Meanwhile, bring the water to a boil in a small saucepan.

- Stir in the quinoa and reduce the heat to medium-low.

- Cook the quinoa for about 15-20 minutes, until it is tender and the water has been absorbed.

- Serve the chicken and vegetable skewers with a side of quinoa and fruit.

# Grilled tofu with roasted vegetables and brown rice

**Description:** This vegan and protein-packed meal features grilled tofu and roasted vegetables served over a bed of nutritious brown rice. It is a great option for a healthy and satisfying dinner.

**Preparation time:** 20 minutes

**Cook time:** 30 minutes

**Ingredients:**

- 1 pound tofu, cut into 1-inch cubes
- 1 bell pepper, cut into 1-inch pieces
- 1 onion, cut into 1-inch pieces
- 1 zucchini, cut into 1-inch pieces
- 1 cup brown rice
- 2 cups water

**Preparation:**

- Preheat the grill to medium-high heat.

- Grill the tofu for about 8-10 minutes, turning occasionally, until it is browned and crispy.

- Meanwhile, preheat the oven to 400 degrees F.

- Toss the vegetables with olive oil and season with salt and pepper.

- Roast the vegetables for about 20-25 minutes, until they are tender.

- Meanwhile, bring the water to a boil in a small saucepan.

- Stir in the brown rice and reduce the heat to medium-low.

- Cook the rice for about 35-40 minutes, until it is tender and the water has been absorbed.

- Serve the grilled tofu with the roasted vegetables and brown rice.

# Dinner recipes to end the day on a healthy note

## Slow cooker turkey chili

**Description:** This hearty and flavorful turkey chili is made in the slow cooker, making it an easy and convenient meal. It's packed with protein, fiber, and a variety of vegetables, making it a healthy and satisfying option for dinner.

**Preparation time:** 15 minutes

**Cook time:** 6-8 hours (in the slow cooker)

**Ingredients:**

- 1 pound ground turkey

- 1 onion, chopped

- 1 bell pepper, chopped

- 1 jalapeno pepper, seeded and minced (optional)

- 1 can (14.5 ounces) diced tomatoes

- 1 can (15 ounces) kidney beans, rinsed and drained

- 1 can (15 ounces) black beans, rinsed and drained

- 1 cup chicken broth

- 1 tablespoon chili powder

- 1 teaspoon ground cumin

- 1/2 teaspoon salt

- 1/4 teaspoon black pepper

- 1/4 cup chopped fresh cilantro

**Preparation:**

- In a large skillet, cook the ground turkey, onion, bell pepper, and jalapeno pepper over medium heat until the turkey is browned and the vegetables are tender.

- Transfer the mixture to a slow cooker.

- Stir in the tomatoes, kidney beans, black beans, chicken broth, chili powder, cumin, salt, and black pepper.

- Cover and cook on low for 6-8 hours.

- Stir in the cilantro before serving.

# Grilled salmon with roasted vegetables

**Description:** This healthy and delicious meal features grilled salmon and a variety of roasted vegetables. The salmon is a rich source of protein and omega-3 fatty acids, while the vegetables provide a variety of nutrients and fiber.

**Preparation time:** 15 minutes

**Cook time:** 20-25 minutes

**Ingredients:**

- 4 salmon fillets
- 1 tablespoon olive oil
- 1/2 teaspoon salt
- 1/4 teaspoon black pepper
- 1 pound mixed vegetables (such as zucchini, bell peppers, and cherry tomatoes)
- 1 tablespoon olive oil
- 1/2 teaspoon salt

- 1/4 teaspoon black pepper

**Preparation:**

- Preheat the grill to medium-high heat.
- Brush the salmon fillets with olive oil and sprinkle with salt and pepper.
- Grill the salmon for 6-8 minutes on each side, or until it is cooked to your desired level of doneness.
- While the salmon is grilling, preheat the oven to 425 degrees F.
- Toss the vegetables with olive oil, salt, and pepper.
- Spread the vegetables on a baking sheet and roast in the preheated oven for 20-25 minutes, or until they are tender and caramelized.
- Serve the grilled salmon with the roasted vegetables.

# Quinoa and Black Bean Salad

**Description:** This hearty and nutritious salad combines the protein-rich grains of quinoa with the fiber and protein of black beans, making it a satisfying and filling meal. It's also packed with vegetables and can be easily customized with your favorite herbs and spices.

**Preparation time:** 10 minutes

**Cook time:** 20 minutes

**Ingredients:**

- 1 cup quinoa, rinsed and drained

- 2 cups water

- 1 can black beans, rinsed and drained

- 1 cup chopped vegetables (such as bell peppers, tomatoes, and cucumbers)

- 1/4 cup chopped fresh herbs (such as cilantro, parsley, and basil)

- 2 tablespoons olive oil

- 1 tablespoon lemon juice

- Salt and pepper to taste

**Preparation:**

- In a medium saucepan, bring the water to a boil. Add the quinoa and reduce the heat to medium-low.

- Cover the saucepan and simmer for about 15-20 minutes, or until the quinoa is tender and the water has been absorbed.

- Remove the saucepan from the heat and let the quinoa cool.

- In a large bowl, combine the cooked quinoa, black beans, vegetables, and herbs.

- In a small bowl, whisk together the olive oil, lemon juice, salt, and pepper. Pour the dressing over the quinoa mixture and toss to combine.

- Serve the salad chilled or at room temperature.

# Baked Chicken with Sweet Potato and Green Beans

**Description:** This flavorful and easy baked chicken dish is paired with tender sweet potatoes and crisp green beans, making it a complete and satisfying meal.

**Preparation time:** 10 minutes

**Cook time:** 35-40 minutes

**Ingredients:**

- 4 chicken breasts
- 1 large sweet potato, peeled and diced
- 1 cup green beans, trimmed
- 1 tablespoon olive oil
- 1 teaspoon paprika
- 1/2 teaspoon garlic powder
- 1/4 teaspoon salt
- 1/4 teaspoon black pepper

**Preparation:**

- Preheat the oven to 400°F.

- In a small bowl, mix together the olive oil, paprika, garlic powder, salt, and pepper.

- Place the chicken breasts in a baking dish and brush them with the olive oil mixture.

- Add the sweet potatoes and green beans to the baking dish, tossing them with the remaining olive oil mixture.

- Bake the chicken and vegetables for 35-40 minutes, or until the chicken is cooked through and the vegetables are tender.

- Remove the baking dish from the oven and serve the chicken and vegetables hot.

Shrimp and broccoli stir-fry

**Description:** This stir-fry is a quick and easy meal that is packed with protein and vegetables. It's a great way to get your daily serving of vegetables in a delicious and flavorful way.

**Preparation time:** 10 minutes

**Cook time:** 15 minutes

**Ingredients:**

- 1 pound shrimp, peeled and deveined

- 2 cups broccoli florets

- 1 tablespoon vegetable oil

- 1 garlic clove, minced

- 1 tablespoon soy sauce

- 1 teaspoon cornstarch

**Preparation:**

- In a small bowl, mix together the soy sauce and cornstarch.

- Heat the oil in a large wok or skillet over high heat.

- Add the broccoli and stir-fry for 2-3 minutes until it is crisp-tender.

- Add the garlic and shrimp and stir-fry for an additional 3-4 minutes until the shrimp are pink and cooked through.

- Stir in the soy sauce mixture and cook for an additional 1-2 minutes until the sauce has thickened.

- Serve hot over rice or noodles.

# Grilled eggplant roll-ups with ricotta and spinach

**Description:** These grilled eggplant roll-ups are a healthy and delicious way to enjoy eggplant. The creamy ricotta and spinach filling adds a delicious flavor and texture to the dish.

**Preparation time:** 10 minutes

**Cook time:** 10 minutes

**Ingredients:**

- 2 medium eggplants, sliced into 1/4 inch rounds

- 1 cup ricotta cheese

- 1 cup chopped spinach

- 1/4 cup grated parmesan cheese

- 1 tablespoon olive oil

- Salt and pepper to taste

**Preparation:**

- Preheat the grill to medium-high heat.

- In a small bowl, mix together the ricotta, spinach, parmesan, and a pinch of salt and pepper.

- Brush the eggplant rounds with olive oil and season with salt and pepper.

- Grill the eggplant rounds for 2-3 minutes on each side until they are tender and have grill marks.

- Spread a spoonful of the ricotta mixture onto each eggplant round and roll up tightly.

- Serve hot.

# Mushroom and Lentil Soup

**Description:** This hearty and flavorful soup combines the rich taste of mushrooms with the protein-rich lentils for a satisfying and nourishing meal.

**Preparation time:** 10 minutes

**Cook time:** 45 minutes

**Ingredients:**

- 1 cup lentils
- 4 cups water
- 1 cup chopped mushrooms
- 1 diced onion
- 2 cloves garlic, minced
- 1 diced carrot
- 1 diced celery stalk
- 1 diced potato
- 1 tsp dried thyme
- 1 tsp dried basil
- 1 tsp salt
- 1/2 tsp pepper

- 1 tbsp olive oil

**Preparation:**

- Heat the olive oil in a large pot over medium heat.

- Add the onion, garlic, carrot, and celery and cook until the vegetables are softened, about 5 minutes.

- Stir in the mushrooms and cook for an additional 5 minutes.

- Add the lentils, water, thyme, basil, salt, and pepper to the pot and bring to a boil.

- Reduce the heat to medium-low and simmer for 30-35 minutes, until the lentils are tender.

- Serve hot.

# Stuffed Bell Peppers with Brown Rice and Ground Turkey

**Description:** These colorful and delicious stuffed bell peppers are filled with a flavorful mixture of brown rice, ground turkey, and vegetables for a satisfying and nutritious meal.

**Preparation time:** 15 minutes

**Cook time:** 45 minutes

**Ingredients:**

- 4 bell peppers, halved and seeded

- 1 cup brown rice

- 2 cups water

- 1 pound ground turkey

- 1 diced onion

- 1 diced bell pepper

- 1 diced tomato

- 1 tsp garlic powder

- 1 tsp onion powder

- 1 tsp paprika

- 1 tsp chili powder

- 1 tsp salt

- 1/2 tsp pepper

- 1 cup shredded cheese (optional)

**Preparation:**

- Preheat the oven to 350°F.

- Cook the brown rice according to package instructions.

- Meanwhile, heat a large skillet over medium heat.

- Add the ground turkey and cook until browned, about 5-7 minutes.

- Stir in the onion, bell pepper, tomato, garlic powder, onion powder, paprika, chili powder, salt, and pepper and cook until the vegetables are tender, about 5-7 minutes.

- Stir in the cooked brown rice.

- Fill the bell pepper halves with the ground turkey and rice mixture and place them in a baking dish.

- Sprinkle the cheese over the top of the stuffed peppers (optional).

- Bake for 20-25 minutes, until the peppers are tender and the filling is heated through.

- Serve hot.

# Grilled vegetables with tofu skewers

**Description:** This delicious and healthy vegetarian dish is perfect for a summer barbecue or a quick and easy dinner. The grilled vegetables and tofu skewers are packed with nutrients and flavor, and they are sure to be a hit with the whole family.

**Preparation time:** 10 minutes

**Cook time:** 20 minutes

**Ingredients:**

- 1 zucchini, sliced into 1-inch rounds
- 1 yellow squash, sliced into 1-inch rounds
- 1 red bell pepper, cut into 1-inch pieces
- 1 onion, cut into 1-inch wedges
- 1 package extra-firm tofu, cut into 1-inch cubes
- 1 tablespoon olive oil
- 1 teaspoon garlic powder
- 1 teaspoon onion powder

- 1 teaspoon dried herbs (such as oregano, basil, or thyme)

- Salt and pepper, to taste

**Preparation:**

- Preheat the grill to medium-high heat.

- In a small bowl, mix together the olive oil, garlic powder, onion powder, and dried herbs.

- Place the zucchini, squash, bell pepper, and onion on a large baking sheet and brush with the olive oil mixture.

- Season with salt and pepper, to taste.

- Thread the tofu onto skewers, alternating with the vegetables.

- Grill the skewers for about 10-12 minutes, turning occasionally, until the vegetables are tender and the tofu is golden brown.

- Serve the skewers hot, with any desired dips or sauces.

# Black Bean and Corn Salad with Avocado Dressing

**Description:** This colorful and flavorful salad is a perfect side dish or main course for a summer picnic or barbecue. The black beans and corn provide protein and fiber, while the avocado dressing adds a creamy and healthy twist.

**Preparation time:** 10 minutes

**Cook time:** 0 minutes

**Ingredients:**

- 1 cup cooked black beans
- 1 cup cooked corn kernels
- 1/2 cup diced tomatoes
- 1/4 cup diced red onion
- 1/4 cup chopped cilantro
- 1 avocado
- 2 tablespoons lime juice
- 1 clove garlic, minced

- 1 teaspoon honey

- Salt and pepper, to taste

**Preparation:**

- In a large bowl, combine the black beans, corn, tomatoes, onion, and cilantro.

- In a small blender or food processor, blend the avocado, lime juice, garlic, honey, and a pinch of salt and pepper until smooth.

- Pour the avocado dressing over the bean and corn mixture and toss to coat.

- Serve the salad chilled or at room temperature.

# Roasted turkey breast with roasted vegetables

**Description:** This flavorful and healthy dinner combines a succulent roasted turkey breast with a variety of nutritious roasted vegetables. The combination of protein and vegetables provides a balanced and satisfying meal.

**Preparation time:** 15 minutes

**Cook time:** 45 minutes

**Ingredients:**

- 1 turkey breast
- 1 cup chopped vegetables (such as carrots, potatoes, and onions)
- 2 tbsp olive oil
- 1 tsp salt
- 1 tsp pepper

**Preparation:**

- Preheat the oven to 375°F.

- Rub the turkey breast with olive oil and season with salt and pepper.

- Arrange the chopped vegetables in a single layer on a baking sheet.

- Drizzle the vegetables with olive oil and season with salt and pepper.

- Place the turkey breast and vegetables in the oven and roast for 45 minutes, or until the turkey is cooked through and the vegetables are tender.

- Remove the turkey breast and vegetables from the oven and slice the turkey breast into thin slices.

- Serve the turkey breast with the roasted vegetables.

# Grilled portobello mushroom burgers

**Description:** These delicious and meatless burgers are made with grilled portobello mushrooms and topped with a variety of flavorful toppings. They are a tasty and healthy alternative to traditional burgers.

**Preparation time:** 10 minutes

**Cook time:** 10 minutes

**Ingredients:**

- 4 portobello mushroom caps
- 4 burger buns
- 1 tbsp olive oil
- 1 tsp salt
- 1 tsp pepper
- Toppings (such as lettuce, tomato, onion, and cheese)

**Preparation:**

- Preheat the grill to medium heat.

- Brush the portobello mushroom caps with olive oil and season with salt and pepper.

- Grill the mushroom caps for 5-7 minutes on each side, or until they are tender and browned.

- Assemble the burgers by placing the grilled mushroom caps on the burger buns and topping with desired toppings.

- Serve the burgers hot.

# Vegetarian Quiche with Whole Wheat Crust

**Description:** This savory and satisfying quiche is filled with a variety of vegetables and topped with a whole wheat crust. It's a delicious and healthy meal that can be enjoyed for breakfast, lunch, or dinner.

**Preparation time:** 15 minutes

**Cook time:** 45 minutes

**Ingredients:**

- 1/2 cup whole wheat flour
- 1/2 cup all-purpose flour
- 1/4 cup cold butter, cut into small pieces
- 1/4 cup cold water
- 1/4 cup chopped vegetables (such as onions, peppers, and mushrooms)
- 1/4 cup shredded cheese (such as cheddar or mozzarella)
- 1/4 cup milk

- 3 eggs

- 1/4 tsp salt

- 1/4 tsp pepper

**Preparation:**

- Preheat the oven to 375°F.

- In a large mixing bowl, combine the flours and butter. Use a fork or your fingers to mix the ingredients until the mixture resembles coarse sand.

- Stir in the cold water until the dough comes together. Press the dough into a 9-inch pie dish.

- In a small mixing bowl, whisk together the eggs, milk, salt, and pepper.

- Scatter the chopped vegetables and shredded cheese over the pie crust. Pour the egg mixture over the top.

- Bake the quiche for 35-45 minutes, or until the crust is golden brown and the eggs are set. Remove the quiche from the oven and let it cool for a few minutes before

serving.

# Grilled Chicken with Roasted Sweet Potato and Asparagus

**Description:** This flavorful and hearty meal features succulent grilled chicken, tender roasted sweet potatoes, and crisp asparagus. It's a perfect combination of protein, carbohydrates, and vegetables.

**Preparation time:** 15 minutes

**Cook time:** 35 minutes

**Ingredients:**

- 4 chicken breasts
- 1 lb sweet potatoes, peeled and cut into 1-inch cubes
- 1 lb asparagus, trimmed
- 2 tbsp olive oil
- 1 tsp garlic powder
- 1 tsp paprika
- 1 tsp salt

- 1/2 tsp pepper

**Preparation:**

- Preheat the grill to medium-high heat.

- In a small mixing bowl, combine the olive oil, garlic powder, paprika, salt, and pepper. Brush the chicken breasts with the seasoning mixture.

- Place the chicken on the grill and cook for 6-8 minutes on each side, or until it reaches an internal temperature of 165°F.

- Meanwhile, place the sweet potato cubes in a single layer on a baking sheet. Roast the sweet potatoes in the oven at 375°F for 20-25 minutes, or until they are tender.

- Meanwhile, toss the asparagus with a little olive oil and place it on the grill. Grill the asparagus for 3-4 minutes on each side, or until it is tender and slightly charred.

- Serve the grilled chicken with the roasted sweet potatoes and grilled asparagus.

# Slow cooker vegetable and bean stew

**Description:** This slow cooker vegetable and bean stew is a hearty and nourishing meal that is easy to prepare and perfect for a cold day. It is packed with a variety of vegetables and beans, making it a great source of plant-based protein and nutrients.

**Preparation time:** 15 minutes

**Cook time:** 8 hours

**Ingredients:**

- 1 cup dried beans (such as kidney, pinto, or black beans)
- 1 cup diced carrots
- 1 cup diced celery
- 1 cup diced onions
- 1 cup diced bell peppers
- 1 cup diced sweet potatoes
- 1 cup diced tomatoes
- 4 cups vegetable broth

- 1 tsp chili powder

- 1 tsp cumin

- 1 tsp paprika

- 1 tsp oregano

**Preparation:**

- Soak the dried beans in water for at least 4 hours or overnight.

- Drain and rinse the beans, then place them in a slow cooker.

- Add the carrots, celery, onions, bell peppers, sweet potatoes, and tomatoes to the slow cooker.

- Pour in the vegetable broth and stir in the chili powder, cumin, paprika, and oregano.

- Cover the slow cooker and cook on low heat for 8 hours or until the beans and vegetables are tender.

- Serve the stew hot, garnished with fresh herbs or a sprinkle of cheese if desired.

# Black bean and quinoa bowls with avocado salsa

**Description:** These black bean and quinoa bowls are a healthy and flavorful meal that is perfect for lunch or dinner. The combination of black beans and quinoa provides a balance of protein and carbohydrates, and the avocado salsa adds a creamy and refreshing element.

**Preparation time:** 15 minutes

**Cook time:** 20 minutes

**Ingredients:**

- 1 cup quinoa
- 2 cups water
- 1 cup cooked black beans
- 1 cup diced tomatoes
- 1 cup diced cucumbers
- 1/2 cup diced red onions
- 1/2 cup diced bell peppers

- 1 avocado

- 1 tbsp lime juice

- 1 tsp chili powder

- 1 tsp cumin

- 1 tsp paprika

**Preparation:**

- Rinse the quinoa in a fine mesh strainer and drain.

- Bring the water to a boil in a small saucepan over medium-high heat.

- Stir in the quinoa and reduce the heat to low.

- Cover the saucepan and cook the quinoa for about 20 minutes, or until the water is absorbed and the quinoa is tender.

- While the quinoa is cooking, mash the avocado in a small bowl and stir in the lime juice, chili powder, cumin, and paprika.

- When the quinoa is done, divide it into bowls and top with the black beans, tomatoes, cucumbers, red onions, and bell peppers.

- Serve the bowls with the avocado salsa on top or on the side.

# Grilled Shrimp and Vegetable Skewers

**Description:** These flavorful skewers combine tender grilled shrimp with a variety of colorful vegetables for a healthy and delicious meal.

**Preparation time:** 20 minutes

**Cook time:** 10 minutes

**Ingredients:**

- 1 pound large shrimp, peeled and deveined
- 1 red bell pepper, cut into 1-inch pieces
- 1 yellow bell pepper, cut into 1-inch pieces
- 1 zucchini, cut into 1-inch pieces
- 1 red onion, cut into 1-inch pieces
- 1/4 cup olive oil
- 2 tablespoons lemon juice
- 1 clove garlic, minced
- 1 teaspoon dried oregano

- 1/2 teaspoon salt

- 1/4 teaspoon black pepper

**Preparation:**

- Soak wooden skewers in water for at least 20 minutes to prevent burning.

- Thread the shrimp and vegetables onto the skewers, alternating between each type.

- In a small bowl, whisk together the olive oil, lemon juice, garlic, oregano, salt, and pepper.

- Brush the skewers with the marinade on all sides.

- Preheat a grill to medium-high heat. Grill the skewers for 5-7 minutes on each side, until the shrimp are pink and the vegetables are tender.

# Spaghetti Squash with Turkey Meatballs

**Description:** This light and healthy meal combines tender spaghetti squash with protein-rich turkey meatballs, making it a perfect choice for a satisfying dinner.

**Preparation time:** 20 minutes

**Cook time:** 45 minutes

**Ingredients:**

- 1 medium spaghetti squash
- 1 pound ground turkey
- 1/2 cup bread crumbs
- 1 egg
- 1/4 cup chopped parsley
- 1 clove garlic, minced
- 1 teaspoon dried basil
- 1/2 teaspoon salt
- 1/4 teaspoon black pepper

- 1 jar marinara sauce

**Preparation:**

- Preheat the oven to 400°F.

- Cut the spaghetti squash in half lengthwise and scoop out the seeds. Place the squash cut-side down on a baking sheet and roast for 40-45 minutes, until tender.

- While the squash is cooking, mix together the ground turkey, bread crumbs, egg, parsley, garlic, basil, salt, and pepper in a large bowl. Form the mixture into small meatballs.

- Heat a large skillet over medium heat and add the marinara sauce. Add the meatballs and simmer for 8-10 minutes, until cooked through.

- Using a fork, scrape the spaghetti squash to create long strands. Divide the squash between serving plates and top with the meatballs and marinara sauce.

# Roasted salmon with roasted vegetables:

**Description:** This healthy and flavorful meal combines succulent roast salmon with a variety of colorful and nutritious vegetables. The salmon provides a good source of protein and omega-3 fatty acids, while the vegetables add fiber, vitamins, and minerals to the dish.

**Preparation time:** 10 minutes

**Cook time:** 30 minutes

**Ingredients:**

- 1 pound salmon fillets
- 1 cup chopped vegetables (such as bell peppers, onions, and zucchini)
- 1 tablespoon olive oil
- 1 teaspoon salt
- 1/2 teaspoon black pepper

**Preparation:**

- Preheat the oven to 400 degrees F.

- Arrange the salmon fillets and vegetables in a single layer on a baking sheet.

- Drizzle the olive oil over the top and sprinkle with salt and pepper.

- Roast the salmon and vegetables for about 25-30 minutes, until the salmon is cooked through and the vegetables are tender and caramelized.

- Serve the roast salmon and vegetables hot, with a sprinkle of chopped herbs or a squeeze of lemon juice, if desired.

# Quinoa and black bean burrito bowls:

**Description:** These tasty burrito bowls are packed with protein, fiber, and complex carbohydrates, making them a satisfying and nourishing meal. The combination of quinoa, black beans, and vegetables creates a flavor-packed and nutrient-rich dish that can be served with a variety of toppings and sauces.

**Preparation time:** 10 minutes

**Cook time:** 20 minutes

**Ingredients:**

- 1 cup quinoa, rinsed and drained
- 1 cup water
- 1 cup canned black beans, rinsed and drained
- 1 cup chopped vegetables (such as tomatoes, onions, and bell peppers)
- 1 tablespoon olive oil
- 1 teaspoon ground cumin

- 1/2 teaspoon salt

- 1/4 teaspoon black pepper

**Preparation:**

- Bring the water to a boil in a small saucepan over medium-high heat.

- Stir in the quinoa, reduce the heat to low, and cover the saucepan with a lid.

- Simmer the quinoa for about 15-20 minutes, until it is cooked and the water is absorbed.

- Meanwhile, heat the olive oil in a large skillet over medium-high heat.

- Add the black beans, vegetables, cumin, salt, and pepper to the skillet and cook, stirring occasionally, until the vegetables are tender and the black beans are heated through.

- Remove the skillet from the heat and stir in the cooked quinoa.

- Divide the quinoa and black bean mixture into bowls and serve with your choice of toppings and sauces, such as diced avocado, salsa, and sour cream.

# Snack recipes to keep you satisfied between meals

## Apple slices with almond butter

**Description:** This simple and healthy snack combines the sweetness of apple slices with the creamy and nutty flavor of almond butter. It's a great way to get a boost of energy and protein in the middle of the day.

**Preparation time:** 5 minutes

**Ingredients:**

- 1 apple, thinly sliced
- 2 tablespoons almond butter
- Preparation:
- Slice the apple into thin wedges or rounds.
- Spread a small amount of almond butter onto each slice of apple.
- Serve and enjoy.

# Hard-boiled eggs with avocado

**Description:** This protein-packed breakfast or snack combines the creamy texture of avocado with the rich flavor of hard-boiled eggs. It's a delicious and nourishing way to start the day or fuel up during the afternoon.

**Preparation time:** 10 minutes

**Cook time:** 10 minutes

**Ingredients:**

- 2 eggs

- 1 avocado

**Preparation:**

- Place the eggs in a small saucepan and cover with cold water. Bring the water to a boil over high heat.

- Once the water reaches a boil, reduce the heat to medium-low and simmer for 10 minutes.

- Drain the eggs and place them in a bowl of ice water to cool.

- Peel the eggs and slice them in half lengthwise.

- Scoop out the avocado and mash it with a fork.

- Divide the avocado onto the egg halves, and serve.

# Greek Yogurt with Berries and Chia Seeds

**Description:** This refreshing snack is full of protein and antioxidants, and it's perfect for satisfying hunger between meals.

**Preparation time:** 5 minutes

**Cook time:** 0 minutes

**Ingredients:**

- 1 cup Greek yogurt

- 1 cup mixed berries (such as strawberries, blueberries, and raspberries)

- 1 tbsp chia seeds

**Preparation:**

- Place the Greek yogurt in a bowl.

- Top with the mixed berries and sprinkle with chia seeds.

- Serve and enjoy.

# Hummus with Carrot Sticks and Celery

**Description:** This simple and satisfying snack is high in fiber and protein, and it's a great way to get in some healthy vegetables between meals.

**Preparation time:** 10 minutes

**Cook time:** 0 minutes

**Ingredients:**

- 1 cup hummus
- 2 carrots, cut into sticks
- 2 celery stalks, cut into sticks

**Preparation:**

- Spread the hummus on a plate.
- Arrange the carrot and celery sticks around the plate.
- Serve and enjoy.

# Turkey Roll-Ups with Lettuce and Mustard

**Description:** These quick and easy roll-ups are a healthy and satisfying snack that is packed with protein and nutrients. The combination of turkey, lettuce, and mustard adds flavor and texture to this snack.

**Preparation time:** 5 minutes

**Cook time:** N/A

**Ingredients:**

- 4 slices of turkey deli meat

- 4 lettuce leaves

- 2 tablespoons mustard

**Preparation:**

- Lay out the slices of turkey on a flat surface.

- Spread a thin layer of mustard on each slice of turkey.

- Place a lettuce leaf on top of each slice of turkey.

- Roll the turkey, lettuce, and mustard into a tight roll-up.

- Slice the roll-ups into bite-sized pieces and serve.

# Edamame with Sea Salt

**Description:** This simple and delicious snack is a great source of protein and fiber. The edamame is lightly seasoned with sea salt, adding flavor and crunch to this snack.

**Preparation time:** 5 minutes

**Cook time:** 10 minutes

**Ingredients:**

- 1 cup frozen edamame
- 1 teaspoon sea salt

**Preparation:**

- Bring a small pot of water to a boil over high heat.
- Add the edamame to the boiling water and cook for about 10 minutes, or until the edamame is tender.
- Drain the edamame and toss with the sea salt.
- Serve the edamame hot or cold as a snack.

# Quinoa and Bean Salad with Vegetables

**Description:** This hearty and flavorful salad is a great source of protein and fiber, and it's packed with colorful vegetables for added nutrients and flavor.

**Preparation time:** 15 minutes

**Cook time:** 15 minutes

**Ingredients:**

- 1 cup quinoa, rinsed
- 1 cup water
- 1 can black beans, drained and rinsed
- 1 cup diced vegetables (such as bell peppers, tomatoes, and onions)
- 1/4 cup chopped fresh herbs (such as cilantro and parsley)
- 1/4 cup lemon juice
- 2 tablespoons olive oil
- Salt and pepper to taste

**Preparation:**

- Bring the water to a boil in a small saucepan over medium-high heat.

- Stir in the quinoa and reduce the heat to medium-low.

- Cover the saucepan and cook the quinoa for about 15 minutes, or until it is tender and the water has been absorbed.

- Remove the saucepan from the heat and let the quinoa cool for a few minutes.

- Meanwhile, in a large bowl, combine the black beans, vegetables, and herbs.

- Stir in the cooled quinoa, lemon juice, and olive oil.

- Season the salad with salt and pepper to taste.

- Serve the salad at room temperature or chilled.

# Tofu and Vegetable Skewers with a Peanut Sauce

**Description:** These flavorful and satisfying skewers are perfect for grilling or roasting, and they're served with a delicious and creamy peanut sauce for dipping.

**Preparation time:** 20 minutes

**Cook time:** 20 minutes

**Ingredients:**

- 1 pound firm tofu, cut into 1-inch cubes

- 1 red bell pepper, cut into 1-inch pieces

- 1 yellow bell pepper, cut into 1-inch pieces

- 1 zucchini, cut into 1-inch slices

- 1/2 cup peanut butter

- 1/4 cup soy sauce

- 2 tablespoons honey

- 2 cloves garlic, minced

- 1/4 teaspoon red pepper flakes

**Preparation:**

- Preheat the grill or oven to medium-high heat.

- Thread the tofu and vegetables onto skewers, alternating the ingredients.

- In a small bowl, whisk together the peanut butter, soy sauce, honey, garlic, and red pepper flakes to make the peanut sauce.

- Brush the skewers with the peanut sauce and place them on the grill or in the oven.

- Cook the skewers for about 10-12 minutes, turning occasionally, until the tofu is golden brown and the vegetables are tender.

- Serve the skewers hot, with the peanut sauce on the side for dipping.

# Kale Chips with Parmesan and Garlic

**Description:** These crispy and flavorful kale chips make for a delicious and healthy snack that is perfect for satisfying those mid-day cravings.

**Preparation time:** 10 minutes

**Cook time:** 20 minutes

**Ingredients:**

- 1 bunch kale, washed and dried

- 2 tablespoons olive oil

- 1/4 cup parmesan cheese, grated

- 1 garlic clove, minced

- 1 teaspoon salt

**Preparation:**

- Preheat the oven to 350°F.

- Tear the kale into bite-sized pieces and place them in a large bowl.

- In a separate small bowl, mix together the olive oil, parmesan cheese, garlic, and salt.

- Pour the mixture over the kale and toss to evenly coat.

- Spread the kale evenly on a baking sheet lined with parchment paper.

- Bake for 15-20 minutes, or until the kale is crispy and the edges are slightly browned.

- Allow the kale chips to cool before serving.

# Cucumber and Hummus Sandwiches

**Description:** These refreshing and protein-packed sandwiches are a quick and easy snack that is perfect for satisfying hunger on the go.

**Preparation time:** 10 minutes

**Cook time:** 0 minutes

**Ingredients:**

- 1 cucumber, sliced into rounds

- 1/2 cup hummus

- 4 slices bread

**Preparation:**

- Spread the hummus evenly on two of the slices of bread.

- Top with the sliced cucumber rounds.

- Cover with the remaining slices of bread to form sandwiches.

- Cut the sandwiches into quarters and serve.

# Smoothie with protein powder and vegetables

**Description:** This refreshing smoothie is a quick and easy way to get your protein and veggies in for the day. It's a great post-workout snack or a quick breakfast on the go.

**Preparation time:** 5 minutes

**Cook time:** 0 minutes

**Ingredients:**

- 1 cup unsweetened almond milk
- 1/2 banana
- 1/2 cup frozen mixed berries
- 1/2 cup chopped spinach or kale
- 1 scoop vanilla protein powder

**Preparation:**

- Place all ingredients in a blender and blend until smooth.

    Pour into a glass and enjoy.

# Mixed nuts and dried fruit

**Description:** This snack is a perfect combination of healthy fats, protein, and natural sweetness. It's a great way to satisfy hunger between meals and keep your energy levels up.

**Preparation time:** 5 minutes

**Cook time:** 0 minutes

**Ingredients:**

- 1/2 cup mixed nuts (such as almonds, cashews, and peanuts)
- 1/4 cup dried fruit (such as raisins, cranberries, or apricots)
- Preparation:
- Combine the nuts and dried fruit in a small bowl or bag. Enjoy as a snack anytime throughout the day.

# Turkey and Cheese Pinwheels

**Description:** These tasty and easy-to-make pinwheels are a great snack or lunch option, and they are packed with protein from the turkey and cheese.

**Preparation time:** 10 minutes

**Cook time:** 10 minutes

**Ingredients:**

- 1/2 cup cooked and diced turkey
- 1/2 cup shredded cheese (such as cheddar or mozzarella)
- 2 large tortillas
- 1/4 cup diced vegetables (such as bell peppers, onions, or spinach)
- 1/4 cup diced avocado

**Preparation:**

- Preheat the oven to 375°F.

- Spread the turkey, cheese, and vegetables evenly over the tortillas.

- Roll the tortillas tightly and cut into 1-inch slices.

- Arrange the slices on a baking sheet and bake for 10 minutes, or until the cheese is melted and the tortillas are crispy.

- Serve the pinwheels warm, garnished with diced avocado if desired.

# Grilled Zucchini with Feta Cheese

**Description:** This simple and flavorful side dish is perfect for summer grilling, and it pairs well with a variety of main courses.

**Preparation time:** 5 minutes

**Cook time:** 10 minutes

**Ingredients:**

- 2 medium zucchini, sliced into rounds
- 1 tablespoon olive oil
- 1/2 teaspoon salt
- 1/2 teaspoon black pepper
- 1/2 cup crumbled feta cheese
- 1/4 cup chopped fresh herbs (such as basil or parsley)

**Preparation:**

- Preheat the grill to medium-high heat.

- Brush the zucchini rounds with olive oil and season with salt and pepper.

- Grill the zucchini for 5-7 minutes on each side, or until tender and slightly charred.

- Remove the zucchini from the grill and sprinkle with feta cheese and fresh herbs.

- Serve the zucchini warm.

# Avocado and egg toast

**Description:** This simple and flavorful breakfast is a tasty way to start the day. It combines creamy avocado with protein-rich eggs and is served on top of toasted bread.

**Preparation time:** 5 minutes

**Cook time:** 5 minutes

**Ingredients:**

- 1 slice of bread
- 1/2 avocado, mashed
- 1 egg
- salt and pepper, to taste

**Preparation:**

- Toast the bread in a toaster or on a pan over medium heat until it is golden brown.
- Spread the mashed avocado over the toasted bread.

- Crack the egg into a small pan and cook over medium heat until the white is cooked and the yolk is at your desired level of doneness.

- Season with salt and pepper.

- Place the cooked egg on top of the avocado toast and serve.

# Overnight oats with nuts and fruit

**Description:** This healthy and convenient breakfast is made by soaking oats in milk overnight, allowing them to soften and absorb the flavors of the other ingredients. It can be customized with your choice of nuts and fruit to add flavor and nutrients.

**Preparation time:** 5 minutes

**Cook time:** 0 minutes (oats are soaked overnight)

**Ingredients:**

- 1/2 cup rolled oats
- 1/2 cup milk (dairy or non-dairy)
- 1/4 cup chopped nuts or seeds (such as almonds, walnuts, or sunflower seeds)
- 1/4 cup chopped fruit (such as berries, apples, or bananas)
- 1 tsp honey or maple syrup (optional)

**Preparation:**

- In a small jar or container, combine the oats, milk, nuts, fruit, and honey or maple syrup (if using).

- Stir well to combine and place the jar in the fridge overnight.

- In the morning, the oats will have softened and absorbed the flavors of the other ingredients. Enjoy cold or heat in the microwave.

# Spiced Popcorn

**Description:** This spicy and flavorful snack is a great alternative to traditional salty popcorn, and it can be a tasty way to satisfy your cravings.

**Preparation time:** 5 minutes

**Cook time:** 5 minutes

**Ingredients:**

- 1/2 cup popcorn kernels
- 1 tsp olive oil
- 1 tsp chili powder
- 1/2 tsp cumin
- 1/2 tsp paprika
- 1/4 tsp salt

**Preparation:**

- Heat the olive oil in a large saucepan over medium heat.

- Add the popcorn kernels and stir until they are coated with oil.

- Cover the saucepan and cook for about 3-5 minutes, shaking the pan occasionally, until the popcorn is popped.

- Remove the saucepan from the heat and sprinkle the chili powder, cumin, paprika, and salt over the popcorn.

- Stir until the spices are evenly distributed.

- Serve the spiced popcorn in bowls or bags.

# Chocolate Protein Balls with Rolled Oats and Nuts

**Description:** These delicious and healthy snacks are packed with protein, fiber, and healthy fats, and they are a great way to fuel your body on the go.

**Preparation time:** 10 minutes

**Cook time:** None

**Ingredients:**

- 1 cup rolled oats

- 1/2 cup protein powder (such as whey or plant-based)

- 1/2 cup chopped nuts or seeds (such as almonds, walnuts, or sunflower seeds)

- 1/2 cup chocolate chips

- 1/2 cup honey or maple syrup

- 1/4 cup coconut oil, melted

- 1 tsp vanilla extract

**Preparation:**

- In a large mixing bowl, combine the rolled oats, protein powder, nuts, and chocolate chips.

- In a small mixing bowl, whisk together the honey, coconut oil, and vanilla extract.

- Pour the wet mixture into the dry mixture and stir until well combined.

- Use a small cookie scoop or spoon to roll the mixture into balls.

- Place the balls on a baking sheet and refrigerate for at least 30 minutes to set.

- Store the protein balls in an airtight container in the refrigerator for up to a week.

# Chapter 8

## Wrapping Up

n this chapter, we will review the key points covered in the book and provide tips for maintaining progress and staying motivated on your insulin-resistance diet plan. We will also provide resources for further information and support to help you continue on your journey to better health and happiness. By following the strategies and recommendations outlined in this book, you can effectively manage insulin resistance and improve your overall quality of life. With the right tools and support, you can take control of your health and achieve your goals.

# A summary of the key points covered in the book

Throughout the book, we have covered a range of topics related to insulin resistance and how to manage it effectively. Here is a summary of the key points covered:

- What is insulin resistance: Insulin resistance is a condition in which the body's cells become resistant to the effects of insulin, a hormone that helps regulate blood sugar levels. Type 2 diabetes, heart disease, and kidney disease are among the health issues that may result from insulin resistance.

- Risk factors and complications: Insulin resistance can be caused by various risk factors, such as being overweight or obese, having a family history of diabetes, and leading a sedentary lifestyle. Complications of insulin resistance can include high blood sugar levels, high blood pressure, and high cholesterol levels.

- A low-glycemic diet to the rescue: A low-glycemic diet is a dieting plan that focuses on foods that are low on the glycemic index, a ranking system that assesses the effect of various kinds of carbohydrates on blood sugar levels. Foods with a low GI value are absorbed more slowly by the body, which can help keep blood sugar levels stable and reduce the risk of insulin resistance.

- The benefits of a low-glycemic diet: Following a low-glycemic diet has numerous benefits, including improved blood sugar control, weight loss, reduced risk of type 2 diabetes, improved heart health, increased energy levels, and improved mood.

- How to incorporate low-glycemic foods into your meals: There are many delicious and creative ways to incorporate low-glycemic foods into your meals. Some strategies include choosing whole grains instead of refined grains, adding more fruits and vegetables to your meals, including legumes, snacking on nuts and seeds, and choosing lean protein sources.

- Strategies for reducing stress and improving sleep: Reducing stress and improving sleep can help improve insulin sensitivity and reduce the risk of insulin resistance. Some strategies for reducing stress and improving sleep include practicing relaxation techniques, exercising regularly, getting enough sleep, practicing good sleep hygiene, and seeking professional help if needed.

- Meal planning made easy: Meal planning can be a helpful tool for managing insulin resistance and improving overall health. Some tips for making meal planning easy include making a list of your favorite low-glycemic foods, planning for the week ahead, using a meal planning template or app, planning for leftovers, keeping it simple, and working with a healthcare provider and registered dietitian to develop an eating plan that meets your individual needs and goals.

- The basics of meal planning for insulin resistance: When meal planning for insulin resistance, it is important to know your goals, understand the role of carbohydrates, consider portion sizes, plan for meals and snacks, be flexible, and work with a healthcare provider and registered dietitian to develop an eating plan that meets your needs and goals.

By following the strategies and recommendations outlined in this book, you can effectively manage insulin resistance and improve your overall quality of life. By having the necessary resources and assistance, you have the ability to manage your well-being and accomplish your objectives.

## Tips for maintaining progress and staying motivated

Maintaining progress and staying motivated can be challenging, especially when it comes to making changes to your diet and lifestyle. However, with the right strategies and support, you can stay on track and continue to make progress toward your health goals. Here are some tips for maintaining progress and staying motivated:

- Set achievable goals: Setting realistic, achievable goals is important for maintaining progress and staying motivated. Ensure that your goals are specific, quantifiable, achievable, meaningful, and have a deadline. This will assist you in maintaining your focus and enthusiasm.

- Keep track of your progress: Keep track of your progress by monitoring key metrics, such as weight, blood sugar levels, and blood pressure. This can help you see the progress you are making and stay motivated to continue.

- Celebrate your successes: It is important to recognize and celebrate your successes, no matter how big or small. This can help you stay motivated and feel good about your progress.

- Find support: Having a supportive network of people can be helpful for maintaining progress and staying motivated. This could include friends, family, or a support group. It is also important to work with a healthcare provider and a registered dietitian to provide guidance and support on your journey.

- Stay flexible: It is okay to make adjustments to your plan as needed. Try not to be too harsh on yourself if you encounter difficulties or make mistakes. Instead, focus on getting back on track and making progress toward your goals.

- Seek help from professionals: If you are struggling to maintain progress or stay motivated, seeking help from a healthcare provider or mental health professional can be beneficial. They can offer assistance and direction to assist you in remaining focused and reaching your objectives.

By following these tips and being consistent with your efforts, you can maintain progress and stay motivated on your insulin-resistance diet plan. By utilizing the necessary tools and receiving proper support, you have the ability to assume control of your wellness and accomplish your objectives.

## Resources for further information and support.

There are many resources available for further information and support when it comes to managing insulin resistance and improving overall health. Here are some options to consider:

- Healthcare providers: Your healthcare provider is a valuable resource for information and support when it comes to managing insulin resistance. They can provide guidance on diet, exercise, and medications and help you develop a plan that meets your individual needs and goals.

- Registered dietitians: Registered dietitians are trained professionals who can provide guidance and support when it comes to nutrition and meal planning. They can help you develop a healthy eating plan that meets your needs and goals and provide tips for incorporating low-glycemic foods into your meals.

- Online resources: There are many online resources available for information and support when it comes to managing insulin resistance. Some options include websites, forums, and social media groups focused on insulin resistance, diabetes, and healthy eating.

- Books and articles: There are many books and articles available on insulin resistance, diabetes, and healthy eating that can provide additional information and support. Look for reputable sources and speak with a healthcare professional or registered dietitian before making any changes to your diet or lifestyle based on information from these sources.

- Support groups: Support groups can be a helpful resource for information and support when it comes to managing insulin resistance. These groups can provide a sense of community and offer a place to share experiences and learn from others.

By using these resources and seeking guidance and support from healthcare professionals, you can effectively manage insulin resistance and improve your overall health. Remember that managing insulin resistance is an ongoing process, and it is important to be consistent and make healthy choices a part of your daily routine.

# Free Gift

Join our mailing list today and receive a copy of "**one of our books**" completely free by clicking the link below.

https://www.aoml.online/

Plus you'll be set to get updates on all our hot new releases and offers, so you'll never miss the stories you love.

https://www.aoml.online/